Red Light Therapy

Harness the Power of Revolutionary Photobiomodulation with Red and Near-Infrared Therapy for Peak Performance, Enhanced Recovery, Well-Being, Optimal Health, and Age-Defying Beauty

Julia E. Chatwin, BSc

© Copyright 2023 Julia E. Chatwin - All rights reserved.

The information contained in this book may not be reproduced, duplicated, or transmitted without direct written permission from the author or the publisher. This book is copyright protected. It is only for personal use. You cannot amend, distribute, sell, or use any part or content within this book without the consent of the author or publisher.

This book is intended for educational and informational purposes only. It should not be construed as medical advice or a substitute for consultation with a qualified healthcare professional.

The use of specific products, services, or companies, used as examples in this book, does not constitute a recommendation or endorsement by the author. Any trademarks, brand names, or other registered product names mentioned, or referred to in this book, are the property of their respective owners and are used solely for the purpose of identification and illustration.

1st Edition 2023

All images licensed through depositphotos.com

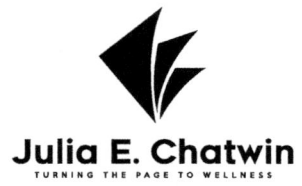

Table of Contents

Introduction 5
About This Book (and why it's for you) 7
Chapter 1 - Red Light Therapy: Background and History 13
Chapter 2 - The Science of Red Light Therapy 29
Chapter 3 - Unveiling the Benefits of Red Light Therapy 51
Chapter 4 - Shedding Light on Safety Concerns 79
Chapter 5 - Getting Practical: What, Where and How 107
Chapter 6 - Using Red Light Therapy at Home 133
Chapter 7 - Even More Things You Need to Know 153
Conclusion 167
Glossary 171

Companion Book

As a way of saying thank you for your purchase, there is a free companion book which I have written called "Discovering the Power of Red-Light Therapy". Join me as I share my personal experience with RLT and the remarkable benefits it has brought to my life. The best part is, I reveal the specific **RLT device I use**—a high quality, yet affordable, entry-level RLT device that has withstood extensive testing, and meets my exacting standards! Perfect for beginners.

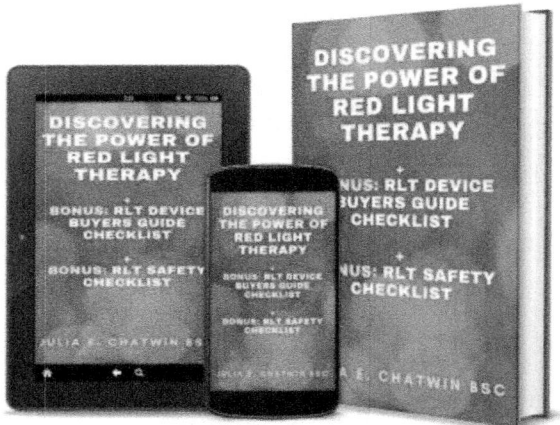

The book also includes two comprehensive 16-point **BONUS** checklists; a compressive RLT Device Buyers Guide Checklist, and an RLT Safety Checklist.

Grab your free copy today, and let the power of red light guide your way to wellness!

https://amitylifebooks.com/rlt

Introduction

"Science is not a collection of facts; it is a process of discovery."
— Robert Zubrin[1]

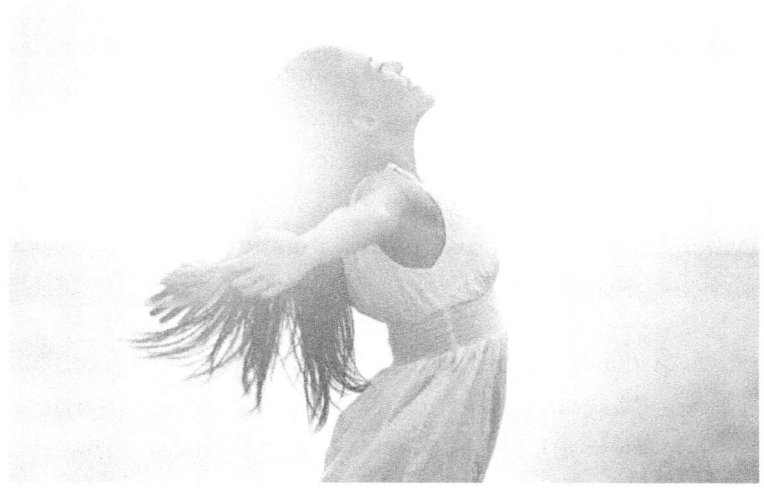

Red light therapy (RLT) is a type of phototherapy (treatment with a special type of light) that uses red low-level lasers or light-emitting diodes (LEDs) to treat various conditions, especially skin conditions. Other names that you might recognise being used to describe red light therapy include low-level laser light therapy (LLLT), low-power laser therapy, soft laser therapy, cold laser therapy, and some non-laser treatments, such as non-thermal LED light, bio stimulation, photonic stimulation, photo bio-modulation, and phototherapy.

RLT is frequently used to lessen pain, reduce inflammation, and promote wound healing after surgery. Seasonal Affective

---

[1] American aerospace engineer and author

Disorder (SAD)—a form of depression that manifests during the winter when there is less natural sunlight, is another condition for which it is occasionally used.

The data suggests that RLT appears to be safe and beneficial for most patients. Negative effects from RLT are infrequent. When they do occur, they are typically minor in nature, such as temporary skin irritation or mild redness. Most of the time, RLT is administered with a hand-held device, or a panel, that sends out red light at a certain wavelength. A treatment session lasts anywhere between five and twenty minutes, depending on the issue being treated.

There is evidence to support the claim that RLT is also effective in treating skin conditions such as acne, rosacea, and psoriasis, to name but a few. RLT has been shown to be helpful for several other conditions, from arthritis to auto-immune disorders. The outcomes are promising. Numerous products are available which are quickly gaining popularity and they are marketed to improve general health and wellness—RLT is becoming very popular indeed!

There are many questions regarding RLT because visible light is a form of electromagnetic radiation. Excessive exposure to specific forms of electromagnetic radiation can pose health risks, for example, to the skin and eyes. As RLT devices emit a lot of red light, some people are concerned that red light might also be harmful if used improperly. As we progress, you will learn everything about how red light therapy works and how it can be used safely.

About This Book (and why it's for you)

Where are you on your journey into the therapeutic applications and benefits of the phototherapy known as red light therapy? You may be well into its use at home, or at a facility. Or you may be new to the subject, and intensely interested in learning more. You may be hoping it can solve a condition that you, or someone you care for, are troubled by; perhaps something that has not responded to traditional medical treatments.

Regardless of where you are on your voyage of discovery, this book contains everything you need to know about red light therapy; whether it's for you; and what you can realistically expect from it.

Like many profound discoveries in life, my introduction to red light therapy came out of a period of personal discomfort and, quite frankly, desperation. To cut a long story short, I suffer from hyperuricaemia. For those that are not familiar, this is a form of inflammatory arthritis, otherwise known as gout.

Now, let me tell you that gout (or the dreaded G word, as I call it), in its infuriating unpredictability, is a formidable opponent. It attacks at the least opportune moments, leaving one in profound pain and crippling discomfort. The intense pain in the affected joints; in my case the knees and feet, can render even the simplest of tasks an excruciating challenge.

I stumbled upon red light therapy out of desperation. I was intrigued by the promising findings from various scientific studies, and driven by an earnest desire to alleviate my gout symptoms, I decided to venture into this novel form of therapy.

Despite the scepticism that naturally accompanies the exploration of alternative therapies, I embarked on this journey with an open mind. I was motivated by the prospect of finding a solution that could not only mitigate my symptoms, but also enhance my overall well-being.

This book is a summation of all that I found. I am sharing the information I found, and the knowledge I gained—both the positive and the negative.

This book gives you full disclosure. Everything will be backed up with science and facts.

Much of what we read about RLT makes it seem to cure everything. But is that true? Are these claims just science fiction? Or is RLT something that has been overlooked and everyone should use it?

The goal of this book is to provide you, the reader, with everything you need to know about RLT and what you can expect from it. You will have many reasons for reading this, and I will attempt to answer all of the questions you may have and help you to use RLT in an informed, responsible manner.

Red light therapy has become an increasingly popular treatment. As a result, it has gained a lot of attention from both medical professionals and wellness enthusiasts alike. In this book, we will explore the science behind red light therapy, its benefits, how it works, and how you can incorporate it into your daily routine to improve your health and well-being. Whether you are a curious newcomer or a seasoned practitioner, this book will provide you with the knowledge and tools to take advantage of the many benefits of red light therapy.

Here's what's inside Red Light Therapy. Below, I summarise what you can expect to learn in each of the book's seven very informative chapters. You can follow the sequence chapter-by-chapter for a solid grounding, or jump ahead if there's a particular subject you are eager to read about. But be sure to cover all of the chapters to become fully knowledgeable about every aspect of RLT.

1. **Red Light Therapy: Background and History:** We begin on a note of caution so you can become alert to all the benefit claims, as well as the safety warnings. You will be able to rely on facts as you make your evaluations and decisions about using RLT. You will learn about the long history of light therapy, how light has influenced evolution, all about wavelengths, the arrival of the laser, and even some space-age experimentation.

2. **The Science of Red Light Therapy:** Here you learn how RLT works, beginning with a quick knowledge-boosting explanation of cellular respiration, and the roles of energy-producing mitochondria and nitric oxide. Then into electromagnetic radiation, and the wavelengths and frequency of light waves in the spectrum. We'll take a first look at the research that has evaluated the effects of RLT, including the benefits at different wavelengths.

3. **Benefits of Red Light Therapy:** The objective is to help you make informed decisions about phototherapy, starting with the Scientific Method, how RLT works, the potential benefits to the skin—treating acne, sun damage, anti-ageing and wrinkles—and healing wounds and scars. We will look at the claims that RLT benefits the hair and scalp, balances hormones, eases pain, relieves arthritis and tendonitis, improves energy, controls dementia and even sexual function.

4. **Shedding Light on Safety Concerns:** We know about the risks of UVA and UVB, but what about red light therapy? We'll cover the importance of protecting your eyes and other precautions, pregnancy risks, cancer cause or cure, hair loss cause or cure, headaches and migraines, and light therapy treatment for seasonal affective disorder.

5. **Getting Practical: What, Where and How:** Locations to receive RLT treatment: the dermatologist's office, other therapy locations, RLT devices to use at home and examples for home use, wearable red light therapy devices, handheld LED devices and red light therapy beds. We the ask the question—are devices purchased for at-home use a safe, reasonable option? (a perspective from the Cleveland Clinic).

6. **Using Red Light Therapy at Home:** Now we're up to the point in the decision-making process where you naturally have questions and concerns that need to be addressed and answered. This chapter is organised into a series of frequently asked questions, which cover the

basics of everything you need to know about safety, the selection of your device, how to operate your device, and other concerns. Then I will summarise mistakes to avoid for optimal, safe results.

7. **Even More Things You Need to Know:** This book is primarily about red light therapy and infrared light therapy, which are at the longest wave, lowest frequency end of the visible segment of the spectrum. But what about the other visible colours of the spectrum? They will be covered here.

So, if you are ready to get started on a thorough presentation of phototherapy, let's get going with Chapter 1's coverage of ancient traditions to modern science.

Julia E. Chatwin

Chapter 1 - Red Light Therapy: Background and History

"Effective health care depends on self-care; this fact is currently heralded as if it were a discovery." — Ivan Illich[2]

From Ancient Tradition to Modern Science

Red light therapy (RLT) applies low-wavelength red light to treat many conditions, from skin disorders to a variety of diseases. In defining RLT, the prestigious Cleveland Clinic (2022) says it "Reportedly improves your skin's appearance, such as reducing wrinkles, scars, redness, and acne. It's also touted to treat other medical conditions."

A Note of Caution

But there's a heads up in that definition; an alert if you are new to RLT, and especially if you have heard or read about its many proclaimed benefits, its safety, and its effectiveness:

- Words like *reportedly* and *touted* are the polite way for a medical authority to say: Not so fast; there's much not yet proven!

Medicine and all of the sciences require **unequivocal**, clinically proven results of extensive testing under controlled conditions before ideas and hypotheses are accepted as fact. We'll get into

---

[2] Theologian, philosopher, and social critic

medical testing protocols and the disciplines of the scientific method a little later on.

But there is **plenty of room for hope** and anticipation of RLT's high potential. An authoritative caution does not and should not diminish the potential benefits, safety, and effectiveness of RLT:

"To date, there's a lot of ongoing research, publication of small studies, and much discussion on the internet about the effectiveness of red light therapy for all types of health uses," the Cleveland Clinic advises. Results of some research do show promise, which is encouraging, "But the full effectiveness of red light therapy has yet to be determined."

This chapter will give you an in-depth background on RLT's origin, early testing, and results. This is all part of the book's objective of helping you make **your own informed decisions** about what it can be used for, what results to expect, and what risks may exist.

Other names that you might recognise being used to describe red light therapy include low-level laser light therapy, low-power laser therapy, soft laser therapy, cold laser therapy. In addition, there are also some non-laser treatments, such as non-thermal LED light, bio stimulation, photonic stimulation, photo bio-modulation, and phototherapy. That's quite a lot to take in. But don't worry, as the book progresses, you will learn more about some of these technologies. We will however be keeping our focus on RLT and its potential for you and for those you care for. After all, that is what the book is all about.

Earliest History

It started with sunlight. Since the dawn of time, humanity has acknowledged and harnessed the therapeutic benefits of light for healing purposes. The earliest records of light therapy go back thousands of years to ancient Egyptian, Greek, and Roman civilisations. Even then, this is where applications of sunlight were used to promote good health and help cure illnesses. We can imagine people enjoying the sunlight in these regions—which tends to have abundant sunshine throughout most of the year. Looking out of the window now, I wish the sun would shine!

The Egyptians were the first to grasp the concept that coloured glass will filter out "All of the other wavelengths of the visible spectrum of light and give you a pure form of red light, which is 600-700 nanometre (nm) wavelength radiation," reports *Red Light Man* (2022). There are records that suggest the early Egyptians (going back to the times of the Pharaohs and pyramids) were advanced enough to construct solariums with coloured glass installed to filter certain colours of the visible spectrum of light to heal disease.

In 1666, known as the *annus mirabilis* or miraculous year, Isaac Newton's scientific experiments with light and prisms led to a new understanding of the properties of light.

Isaac Newton experimented by passing sunlight through prisms, which refracted (bent) the light, and was able to demonstrate that pure white sunlight was composed of seven visible colours: Red, orange, yellow, blue, green, indigo, and violet. He called this phenomenon the light spectrum. In scientific terms, the light spectrum refers to the range of electromagnetic radiation wavelengths that can be detected by the human eye. This is also what is referred to as visible light. The spectrum ranges longer wavelengths, which appear red in colour, to shorter wavelengths, which appear violet in colour.

Beyond the visible spectrum, there are even shorter wavelengths of radiation such as ultraviolet and X-rays, and even longer wavelengths such as infrared and radio waves. We say beyond the visible spectrum because it is just that—the human eye cannot see these types of light.

Each type of electromagnetic radiation has a different wavelength and frequency. They can be used in various applications, from medical imaging to telecommunications. They can even be used to heat your food.

As clever as the Egyptians were, during these early times, any perceived benefits of sunlight would be anecdotal. Benefits would be based on observations, word of mouth, and unproven assumptions. Yet even today, with all that is known about the dangers of sun exposure, how many of us still like a nice tan complexion, and believe it looks and feels healthier? Our dermatologists would most strenuously disagree. What people think, and what science can prove, are often quite different.

Evolutionary Effects

The availability—or lack—of sunshine strongly affected the evolution of skin types, with direct relationships developing between sunlight and skin colour. Races that evolved in warmer regions closer to the equator, where the sunlight is intense, tend to be darker-skinned. People here have a large amount of the colour-providing hormone melatonin, which protects their skin.

In contrast, races that evolved in the colder, more northern regions, which are sun-deficient (less intensive light, and far fewer sunny days), tend to be lighter-skinned. These people lack the protective melatonin—it is not required. This condition makes it easier for their skin to absorb the sparse, beneficial sun's rays. Looking out of the window now, it is very sparse indeed!

When the sun does shine, these people are more susceptible to sunburn and sun-induced skin damage, including skin cancer:

- When people from the sun-deprived north migrate to the south or other sunny regions, they are at exceptional risk. For example, when people of British and Irish descent move to sunny Australia and New Zealand, they need to take precautions that will protect their skin; a worry that does not affect the dark-skinned original peoples of those island nations.

Wavelengths

As mentioned, sunlight is composed of many different wavelengths, from infrared to visible light to ultraviolet. This last light type is composed of two types of rays, UVA and UVB, which has with varying positive and negative effects. It is well known that prolonged exposure to the ultraviolet UVB light as found in sunlight can cause sunburn, skin dehydration (dryness), premature wrinkles, and most significantly, skin cancer. Types of skin cancer are numerous—melanoma, basal cell, and squamous cell carcinomas being common.

UVA is less of a risk, but is known to generate free radicals and damage elastin and collagen in the skin. "UVA partners up with UVB to cause more serious problems, like skin cancer," says dermatologist Saira George, M.D., at the M.D. Anderson Cancer Center (2019).

Yet there are **positive benefits** from sunlight deriving from the effects of ultraviolet light—in moderation, of course, given the downsides just mentioned. This is especially true of the benefits involving vitamin D. UVB rays interacting with cholesterol in the skin contribute to the formation of vitamin D3, which is essential for strong bones and in the prevention of osteoporosis. Studies show that even in northern climates, just a few minutes of the skin's exposure to midday sunlight each day is enough to produce vitamin D. This is without risking skin damage or carcinogenesis.

It was these early experiences with sunlight that led to efforts to isolate light at specific wavelengths that could be beneficial without having negative side effects. These experiments led to the identification of the visible red light part of the spectrum as potentially offering considerable beneficial qualities, with minimal or no risks:

- Studies show that "The red part of the visible light spectrum (600 to 1000 nm) also interacts with a key metabolic enzyme in our cell's mitochondria, raising the lid on our energy generating potential," according to *Red Light Man* (2022).

A Scandinavian Pioneer

Closer to our times, light therapy as a medical practice began in the late 1800s, by which time the industrial revolution and scientific experimentations were in full swing. Electricity had been brought under control and put to practical use, especially in laboratories. At this time, Dr. Niels Ryberg Finsen, a Faroe Islands/Icelandic physician, began experimenting with light as a treatment for disease.

Finsen's work with light therapy was driven by his own disorders: He suffered from Niemann–Pick disease (an inherited metabolic disorder), which "Inspired him to sunbathe and investigate the effects of light on living things". As a result, he created a "Theory of phototherapy, stating that certain wavelengths of light have beneficial medical effects". It's interesting that he sunbathed in a far northern climate with minimal sunlight; at least this lowered his risks of sun damage!

The scientific and medical value of his work with light therapy was recognised in 1903, when Dr. Finsen was awarded the Nobel Prize in Medicine and Physiology, "In recognition of his contribution to the treatment of diseases, especially lupus vulgaris, with concentrated light radiation, whereby he has opened a new avenue for medical science" (*Wikipedia*, 2022). He was the first person from a Scandinavian country to win the prize and was the only Nobel Laureate from the Faroe Islands.

Dr. Kellogg. Following Dr. Finsen's accomplishments, a book entitled *Light Therapeutics* was published in 1910 by no less than Dr. John Harvey Kellogg. Yes, Dr. Kellogg—the American physician and nutritionist who created Kellogg's Corn Flakes and other breakfast cereals.

The book reported the doctor's efforts to heal people with arc lights and more common incandescent light bulbs. His findings conclude that "Light therapy is effective for treating diabetes, obesity, chronic fatigue, insomnia, baldness, cachexia, and many other health problems" (*End All Disease,* 2022).

Enter the Laser

The history of lasers (Light Amplification by Stimulated Emission of Radiation) dates back to the early 20th century, when Albert Einstein proposed the concept of stimulated emission, which forms the basis of laser technology. Some of the first of the more contemporary red light therapy experiments were conducted in 1967 by professor Endre Mester, a Hungarian physician who was studying how cancer cells reacted to electromagnetic radiation exposure. His work was possible due to the invention of the laser in 1960 by American physicist Theodore H. Maiman:

The first working laser, demonstrated by Theodore Maiman in 1960, used a synthetic ruby crystal as the lasing medium. The ruby laser consisted of a rod-shaped ruby crystal, with chromium ions embedded in it, placed between two mirrors. The ruby crystal was optically exposed to a high-energy flash lamp, which excited the chromium ions and caused them to emit photons of light. These photons of light were then amplified by the mirrors and emitted as a narrow, coherent beam of laser light. The ruby laser was a major breakthrough in laser technology.

Following this breakthrough, researchers quickly began developing new types of lasers using different materials as the lasing medium. In 1962, the first gas laser was demonstrated, using a mixture of helium and neon as the lasing medium. This was followed by the development of other gas lasers, including carbon dioxide lasers, which are still widely used today in industrial cutting and welding applications. Although the ruby laser has some limitations, such as limited tunability and low efficiency, it is still used today in some applications, such as in scientific research and in medical procedures.

Throughout the 1960s and 1970s, researchers also developed solid-state lasers using materials such as glass and garnet. These lasers offered greater efficiency and tunability than earlier designs, and were used in a range of applications, including scientific research, telecommunications, and military defence. In the 1980s and 1990s, researchers continued to refine laser technology, developing new types of lasers such as diode lasers and semiconductor lasers, which are now used in everything from barcode scanners to DVD players.

Ruby lasers are still used in some applications, such as in medical procedures and in scientific research, where their high-power output and short pulse durations can be advantageous. Dr. Mester was one of the first to recognise that the laser had significant medical therapeutic value; that its intensity and precision could help to eradicate cancer cells.

He went to work with lasers, but his initial experiments had some unexpected results:

- The experiments directed high-intensity laser beams at cancer cells that had been implanted under the skin. The beams did not appear to destroy the cancer cells but did speed up the healing of the wounds caused by the cell implantation.

- This led to further experiments. This time using low-level lasers which delivered concentrated red and near-infrared light that **proved** that treatment with red light encouraged faster healing of the skin.

- Subsequently, Dr. Mester's other experiments demonstrated that skin defects, venous insufficiency, burns, infected wounds, and diabetes-caused ulcers also healed faster in response to his laser treatment. Light therapy was well on its way.

Space-Age Experimentation

While RLT has been used in various medical and aesthetic applications on Earth, it has also been explored for use in space, particularly by NASA. In fact, not long after the work of Dr. Mester was published, RLT began to be used by NASA in various experiments. In the microgravity environment of space, plants grow differently than they do on Earth, which can impact their development and nutritional content. In these experiments, NASA scientists used red and blue LED lights to provide the necessary light spectrum for plant growth, with the addition of RLT to stimulate cellular activity and promote photosynthesis. The results of these experiments have been promising, with some studies showing that RLT can increase the growth rate and nutritional content of plants grown in space.

In addition to its use in plant growth, RLT is also being explored by NASA for its potential use in treating a range of medical conditions in space, including wound healing, bone loss, and muscle atrophy. RLT has been shown to improve circulation, reduce inflammation, and promote tissue repair, which could make it a valuable tool for maintaining astronaut health during long-duration space missions. The results of these experiments were sufficiently positive to encourage further experimentation with a range of other potential applications of RLT for use by NASA.

Now, let's advance a couple of decades to discover that the work of Dr. Mester had continued in the experiments of his son, Adam Mester. 20 years after his father's laser treatments, he was reported "to have been using lasers to treat 'otherwise incurable' ulcers" (reported in *Cure All Disease*, citing a New Republic article from 1987). It is also cited that "he takes patients referred by other specialists who could do no more for them". The article reads, and reports that Dr. Adam Mester had treated a total of 1,300 patients and "achieved complete healing in 80 per cent and partial healing in 15 percent." These were people who could not be helped by previous treatments. A total of 95 percent were healed or appreciably helped by the application of red laser therapy.

Fast forward to today, and we can record that red light therapy has medical application in a technology called photodynamic therapy (PDT). Photodynamic therapy is not to be confused with "standard" Red Light Therapy. Photodynamic therapy is a type of treatment that uses a **combination** of a photosensitising agent and light (red or otherwise) to destroy cancerous and pre-cancerous cells, as well as some types of bacterial infections. During this procedure, low-power red laser light is directed towards a drug that is sensitive to light waves. As a result, the drug's effects are altered. It is also used to acne cells, cells underlying psoriasis, and warts. PDT is a minimally invasive treatment that is typically performed on an outpatient basis and is less damaging to healthy tissue than other cancer treatments, such as chemotherapy or radiation therapy. In the UK, PDT is used in hospitals and by the National Health Service (NHS) to treat a variety of conditions, including skin cancer, lung cancer, and some types of head and neck cancers.

RLT in various forms is being tested for its effectiveness and safety in many medical conditions. But again, we need to be less accepting and more investigative in deciding that RLT, or indeed in any new treatment, has been fully tested for safety and effectiveness by responsible laboratories. Let us explore further.

A Special Advantage

RLT and other forms of phototherapy are distinguished from many other types of treatment for diseases and medical conditions because light therapy is non-invasive (which means nothing goes inside of you, except for possibly penetrating outer skin cells). Light therapy is also nonchemical, nondrug, nontoxic, and does not apply excessive amounts of heat which can burn or irritate the skin.

Also, RLT does not use ultraviolet (UVA and UVA) light, which eliminates any risk of the negative effects we mentioned in this chapter.

These qualities, in themselves, do not imply or confirm RLT's safety or its effectiveness. In situations where it passes testing scrutiny, it would be potentially more acceptable to patients and considered safe for all skin types.

Intensive Research

As the 21st century got underway, interest in red light therapy and other forms of phototherapy had reached its peak, and was being replaced by other medical practices, from advanced drugs to more effective forms of surgery. Genetic sciences and manipulation of the human genome become the central focus. To many medical and scientific authorities, light therapy in all its versions was suspicious and questionable.

But instead of fading away as an outdated and unreliable form of medical treatment, a renewed interest in red light therapy and all the other forms of phototherapy has emerged. Why? In part, because there has been, all along, evidence of at least some positive results, leading to a determination to conduct better research, under controlled conditions, to learn how to use light therapy effectively and safely. The non-invasive, nontoxic features undoubtedly contribute to the new interest as well.

A 2018 keyword search in the U.S. National Library of Medicine of the different names describing light therapy yields a total of over 50,000 published scientific and clinical studies. Phototherapy accounted for 37,785 of those studies in 2018; it is assuredly much higher today.

Chapter Summary

How do we bring this long history of light therapy to an objective, unbiased conclusion? Here are perspectives for your consideration:

- History is on the side of light therapy. No practice or procedure that offers important health benefits can survive and even flourish for thousands of years. Trends and fads come and go, but there has to be something solid, persistent, and enduring to last that long with at least a portion of the population. Sometimes it takes faith, or trust, just as with spiritual values.

- But belief and enthusiasm are not proof of effectiveness or validation of benefit claims. Even today, we are awash in product performance and benefit claims that are unconfirmed by valid research, including clinical trials.

This is how it should be done: We witnessed the serious, scientific clinical trials that were conducted on the COVID-19 mRNA vaccines before the CDC and FDA gave their approvals. The four-stage trials first tested for safety and concluded with 10,000 participants; a screened, representative sample that is large enough for the results to be statistically significant.

- The existence of scientific proof can help to confirm benefit claims in most cases, but the absence of proof does not mean the benefits are invalid or untrue; it just means they have not yet been validated, and the claims of benefits should not be treated as true.

For example, the need for us to take 10,000 steps a day for fitness is actually a marketing idea from a Japanese pedometer manufacturer; no research was undertaken to validate that target number. In contrast, tests are being conducted to determine, under controlled conditions, if there is a medically valid daily step target. (So far, it's looking like 5,000 to 7,000 steps a day will do the job.)

What's next? This background has brought us from thousands of years ago to the present, so let's focus on what is known today about the science of red light therapy and other phototherapy methods. Don't worry; this will be science written to be understood.

Julia E. Chatwin

Chapter 2 - The Science of Red Light Therapy

"I seem to have been only like a boy playing on the seashore, and diverting myself in now and then finding a smoother pebble or a prettier shell than ordinary, whilst the great ocean of truth lay all undiscovered before me." — Isaac Newton[3]

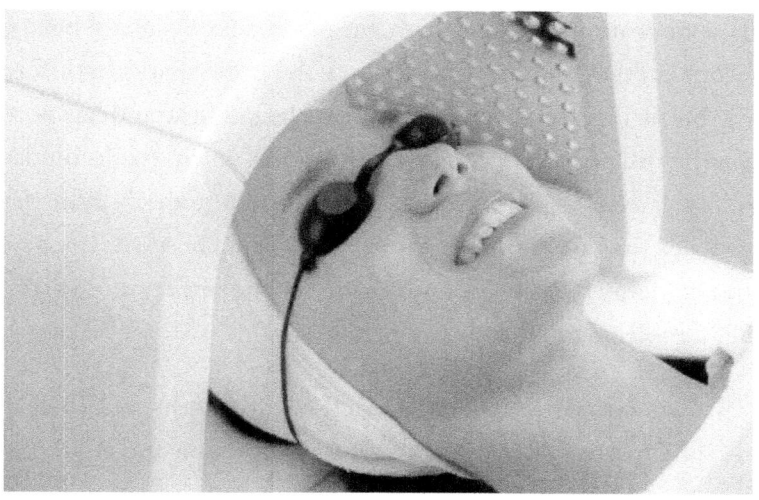

Now that you know what RLT is, you are probably wondering how it works. This chapter will explain the basics to you.

How Red Light Therapy Works

The effects of RLT take place at the cellular level, and cellular activity is mostly at the molecular and even atomic level. For this reason, we will need to talk about biochemistry for a little while. Don't be concerned if you don't immediately grasp some of these

---

[3] English mathematician, physicist and astronomer

submicroscopic interactions. Just by reading through the following, you should get a sense of how your body and metabolism work.

Stick with it—this background will be incredibly helpful as we move through this book.

One of the key players you will be meeting is nitric oxide, a chemical that is important to many biologic processes in the body. It is a neurotransmitter, which means it sends signals between neurons (nerves), and it controls how the brain works in different ways. Nitric oxide also helps to regulate blood flow and has potent anti-inflammatory properties. In the body, nitric oxide binds to *cytochrome c oxidase* (CCO), an enzyme found in mitochondria (tiny organelles that are the powerhouse of cells). These enzymes help convert energy from food sources into adenosine triphosphate, or ATP, a molecule that cells use for energy.

We will get back to nitric oxide in a few paragraphs, but first, let's pause and get to know more about mitochondria and ATP.

Cellular Respiration

If you've wondered how the food you eat and the oxygen you breathe actually go to work for you, imagine this incredible metabolic process that is taking place right now in the trillions of cells in your body so your cells can have the energy they need to make proteins. This is called cellular respiration, and it is the foundation of life:

- The carbohydrates you eat are broken down during digestion from starches and complex sugars into a simple molecule made of carbon, oxygen, and hydrogen; you know it as glucose.

- The glucose passes into your blood, where capillaries bring it to your cells, and it is absorbed and then passes into the mitochondria. But first, enzymes (which are proteins that catalyse, or cause reactions) in the cytoplasm liquid in the cells break down the glucose into even simpler sugars called pyruvates, and also produce two ATP molecules which help fuel the ongoing metabolic process (patience; many more ATP molecules are coming!).

- The pyruvates and other molecules, including *NADH* and *coenzyme* A, then pass into the mitochondria to take part in an amazing process known as the *electron transport chain*, which involves proteins and electrons passing in and out of the mitochondria's inner membrane. (Mitochondria have a double membrane; an outer one to keep out the cytoplasm of the cell and other items, and an inner membrane, where much of the action takes place).

- This protein-pumping process borrows energy from those first two ATP molecules to energise the electrons, which then connect with oxygen molecules (O_2) in the *Krebs Cycle* that help the molecules turn into citric acid (yes, the same stuff in oranges), and finally we end up with 36 (or more) ATP molecules being produced. This represents more stored up energy, ready to be released as needed.

- What is this potent energy storehouse? The ATP molecule is composed of adenosine (a nitrogenous base), ribose (a sugar molecule), and a string of three phosphate molecules (the "tri" of triphosphate), which are held together by high-energy hydrogen bonds.

- It's in these three bonded phosphate molecules where the energy our cells need is stored, and on cue, the ATP kicks off one of its three phosphate molecules, breaking and releasing a high-energy hydrogen bond to form ADP or adenosine diphosphate. That released energy is powering your muscles, your organs, your brain, and especially your heart. (Your heart muscle cells are about 45% composed of mitochondria, compared to 20% to 25% in your other muscles, and only 5% in skeletal tissues).

The reason for this detailed explanation is to help you understand just how important these mitochondria really are, and why red light's influence can be so important. If the wavelengths of red light actually reach the mitochondria and influence their critical operations, that's very important for us to recognise.

The Role of Nitric Oxide

This brings us back to nitric oxide (NO), also called nitrogen monoxide; it's a colourless gas formed by the oxidation of nitrogen. "Nitric oxide performs important chemical signalling functions in humans and other animals" (*Britannica*, 2022). It is essential to the functioning of the mitochondria in our cells, functioning as both an energy producer and metabolic regulator.

Because of its importance in cellular metabolism, nitric oxide is thought to be a potential therapeutic target for treating disorders like diabetes and cardiovascular disease. Nitric oxide affects both crucial functions of mitochondria; the generation of energy and the control of cell death. It does this by modulating the production of reactive oxygen intermediates and of ATP.

Deeper dive. Now we're going deeper into the biochemistry behind all of these critical functions; be patient and give it a read-through, because later on, it will help you to understand how red light therapy operates at the cellular level. You'll be reading about enzymes; you will recall that these are protein molecules that cause chemical reactions between other proteins.

To begin, let's introduce an enzyme called cytochrome c oxidase, or Complex IV, which is a "Large transmembrane protein complex found in bacteria, archaea, and mitochondria of eukaryotes," explains *Wikipedia* (2022). (Eukaryotes are cells that contain a nucleus with DNA, which is fundamental to animal life):

- Complex IV is the "Last enzyme in the respiratory electron transport chain of cells located in the membrane." This means that the enzyme receives one electron from each of four other cytochrome c molecules and "Transfers them to one oxygen molecule (O2) and four protons" (a single proton is a hydrogen atom). This leads to the formation of the familiar molecule, H2O, which is water; there are two hydrogen atoms and one oxygen atom in each water molecule.

- Scientists have long debated over the exact way that nitric oxide attaches to cytochrome c oxidase. Nitric oxide may directly bind to the 'haem group' in red blood cells, which is the non-protein component of oxygen-carrying haemoglobin, located in the middle of the iron-containing active site of the protein, according to one line of evidence.

- Others, however, have proposed that in order for nitric oxide to bind to anything, an intermediary molecule must first bind to the haem group. This intermediate may be another chemical that is involved in cellular metabolism, like an amino acid. Research on this issue is ongoing.

- Despite its importance, nitric oxide can damage cells if levels are too high or if it cannot be properly metabolised. This appears to be the case when cytochrome c oxidase is in contact with excessive nitric oxide. Because it disrupts numerous cellular processes, such as DNA replication and mitochondrial respiration, nitric oxide can kill cells when produced in excess for long periods of time. Low levels of cytochrome c oxidase activity have been associated with several diseases, such as heart disease and chronic fatigue syndrome.

This brings us to how this affects, and is affected by, phototherapy: Red and near-infrared light are thought to be primarily absorbed by cytochrome c oxidase in the body, increasing the bioactivity of nitric oxide. This appears to return this enzyme's levels to normal, upregulating its activity while simultaneously enhancing energy production, cellular health, and general health. The advantages of RLT for other conditions and diseases connected to low cytochrome c oxidase activity require further studies, as research into this promising modality progresses.

You have now completed your primer on the metabolic processes and quick education in biochemistry! Phew!

Summing up, you should now know that phototherapy potentially provides restorative benefits at the **cellular** and **intracellular** levels.

This brings us to the properties and characteristics of the light that is used in phototherapy.

Frequencies and Wavelengths of Light

These two terms—frequency and wavelength—will be showing up often in this and other chapters, so a good grounding on what they mean and why they're important is in order.

Light is part of a wide spectrum of electromagnetic radiation (EMR), which is one of the four known universal forces or energies in what's known in quantum mechanics as the Standard Model. The other three are the force of gravity; the weak force that mediates atomic decay; and the strong force which holds the nucleus of atoms together. Two other forces—dark matter and dark energy—are believed to influence galactic movement but have not yet been positively identified. But that is for another book…

Light is but one form of electromagnetism. It is a fundamental force in nature that encompasses both electricity and magnetism. As the name implies, this force is responsible for the interaction between electric charges and magnetic fields. The unified theory of electromagnetism was established in the latter half of the 19th century by the renowned physicist James Clerk Maxwell. Maxwell's work was built upon the earlier discoveries of several prominent scientists, including Michael Faraday, who made a significant contribution to our understanding of electromagnetism.

The speed of light is 186,282 miles (299,792 km) per second, which means light from the moon (250,000 miles away) takes about 1.3 seconds to get here, and light from the sun (93,000,000 miles from us) takes about 8.2 minutes to arrive. Even at this impressive speed, light from the most distant galaxies that the Hubble and James Webb space telescopes are detecting has been travelling for billions of years to reach their lenses. Nothing can travel faster than light, as Albert Einstein's 1905 Theory of Special Relativity posited, and which has been verified extensively.

Light is a wave, isn't it? Physicists long believed that light travels as a wave, as we would expect. But light can also travel as a particle, which they have named the "photon." Experiments shining a light on a board with parallel slits prove that light may take either form:

- "The double-slit experiment is one of the most famous experiments in physics and definitely one of the weirdest. It demonstrates that matter and energy (such as light) can exhibit both wave and particle characteristics—known as the particle-wave duality of matter" (*Space.com,* 2022).

Today's quantum physicists, while still perplexed, are comfortable with light being a particle when travelling through the vacuum of space. But also, as a light being a wave when passing through the atmosphere, which provides a tangible medium for wavelike activity. Since we're here on Earth, and not en route to Neptune, we'll keep our focus on light waves going forward.

"Light waves have two defining characteristics: wavelength and frequency. Frequency is defined as the number of oscillations of a wave per unit of time, measured in Hertz (Hz); wavelength is defined as the distance between the two most near points in phase with each other. Hence, two adjacent peaks or troughs on a wave are separated by a distance of a single complete wavelength" (*Byjus,*2022).

If that description is hard to visualise, here's a way to picture these characteristics in your mind. Imagine a line extending from left to right, starting at a low point, rising to a crest at the middle, then sinking back down to the starting level when it reaches the right side:

- The low points are called valleys; the high point in the middle is a peak or crest.

- The distance between the peak and the next peak is the wavelength. (It can also be expressed as the distance between a valley and the next valley).

- Frequency is how many peaks (separated by a trough or valley) occur in one second. If a wave oscillates 10,000 times per second, it has a frequency of 10,000 Hertz (Hz).

Since light travels at 186,282 miles per second, the sum of frequency per second multiplied by wavelength is always 186,282.

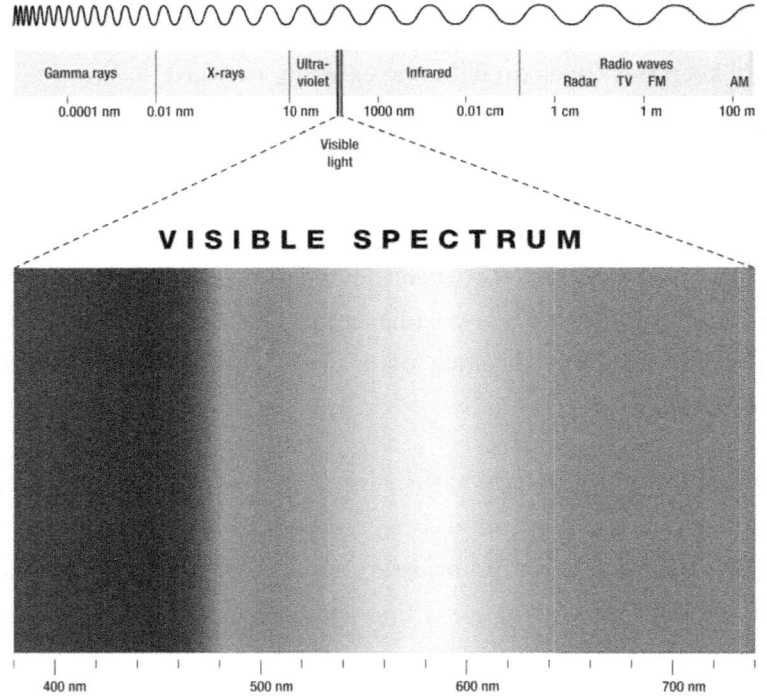

The EMR spectrum is generally shown beginning on the left, with gamma rays and x-rays having the highest frequencies and shortest wavelengths; the spectrum then proceeds to the right with increasingly lower numbers of frequencies and longer wavelengths, culminating with microwaves and radio waves having the lowest frequencies and longest wavelengths:

As you can see, UV light is to the left of visible light, meaning UV has a greater frequency and a shorter wavelength than visible light, and infrared light has a lower frequency but greater wavelength than visible light. Stars—including our sun–emit infrared, visible, and UV light, along with many other forms of radiation. A prism refracts white sunlight into its components based on their wavelengths; we see the colours, but not the infrared and UV, which are invisible to us.

Long-Wavelength Red Light

"Red light occupies the 'therapeutic window' where light emits at a wavelength that will work on our cells without causing damage," notes *Red Light Clinic* (2022). This window extends from about 600 nanometres (nm) to a wavelength of 1200 nm. (A nanometre is one billionth of a metre).

Good to know: ROYGBIV is an acronym that represents the sequence of colours found in a rainbow or in the visible light spectrum. Each letter corresponds to a specific colour. It ordered from the longest wavelength to the shortest wavelength:

- R – Red
- O – Orange
- Y – Yellow
- G – Green
- B – Blue
- I – Indigo

- V - Violet

To avoid confusion caused by the ROYGBIV acronym, the light spectrum begins on the left side (shorter wavelengths) with ultraviolet, then the increasingly longer wavelength visible colours: Violet, indigo, blue, green, yellow, orange, and red, followed by the non-visible, infrared light (longer wavelengths). Perhaps the acronym should be VIBGYOR!

Your eye can see the light of wavelengths between 380 nm (shortest for violet) and 700 nm (longest for red). Although you can't see ultraviolet light, its UVA and UVB rays can burn or damage your skin; and while you can't see infrared light, you can feel its energy as beneficial warmth and heat. It is still going strong after its 93-million-mile journey from the surface of the sun. Infrared light extends from 700 nm (the wavelength where visible red ends) to 1,200 nm, the end of the therapeutic light window.

Propelled By NASA

Expanding on the earlier mention of the role of NASA in testing red light's potential benefits for plants and humans: The potential of red light therapy applications got a big boost when NASA biologists began testing red-light emitting LED lights in the 1990s to affect the growth of plants in gravity-less space.

"Noticing that the plants responded extremely well to the red light (with the longer wavelengths stimulating photosynthesis and causing rapid but healthy growth), scientists began to wonder if they would have a similarly rejuvenating effect on astronauts, who faced many health challenges thanks to prolonged periods of weightlessness" (Red Light Clinic, 2021).

NASA started light therapy trials on astronauts, given the name "WARP" for "Warfighter Accelerated Recovery by Photo bio modulation," and were encouraged by the results, finding that "Red light could provide relief for exhausted and depleted astronauts, treating their arthritis, muscle spasms, and stiffness, as well as increasing blood circulation."

Based on those exceptionally encouraging findings, and the knowledge acquired, NASA began a program of expanded use of red light therapy beyond just astronauts to a range of military applications for frontline soldiers.

Red Light Research

Inspired by the positive results achieved by NASA, numerous studies have been conducted; some recently, to clinically prove (or disprove) the effectiveness of RLT in treating a variety of conditions.

RLT has been adopted enthusiastically by the alternative health community. Its adherents recognise the natural functions of this form of therapy and its gentle stimulation of the body to activate its own self-healing action. This is instead of depending on drugs and medications, or surgical interventions, with their inherent risks.

NASA's WARP technology applied RLT wavelengths of 670 nm, which is in the visible part of the spectrum, but researchers are now testing the benefits of the entire red light range, from 630 nm to 700 nm, just into the edge of infrared light:

- So far, benefits of healing and repair of wounds, pain relief, and anti-inflammatory activities have been observed as a result of applying these extended red light wavelengths. Work is continuing to test these and other wavelengths.

Here are results from additional phototherapy research, which shows positive results for RLT and Low-Level Light Therapy in different medical applications:

Dental

A study was conducted to evaluate the effectiveness of LED red light in the treatment of temporomandibular dysfunction syndrome (TDS), a common dental disease. "It occurs as a consequence of malfunction of the temporomandibular and/or surrounding facial muscles" (NIH, 2019). The study was conducted among 50 students (40 females; 10 males) with TDS.

Results: "The changes in the pain value and number of the tender muscles in both groups were highly significant," though insignificantly lower in the placebo group, leading to the conclusion that "Red LED therapy could be useful in improving patients' symptoms regarding pain, clicking, and number of tender muscles. In addition, this study showed the importance of the psychological part of treatment of those patients."

Skincare

A controlled trial was conducted among 113 subjects and 23 control volunteers to "Determine the efficacy of red and near-infrared light treatment in patient satisfaction, reduction of fine lines, wrinkles, skin roughness, and intradermal collagen density increase" (NIH, 2014).

Results: The treated patients had significantly improved (vs. control) "skin complexion and skin feeling, profilometrically assessed skin roughness, and ultra-sonographically measured collagen density." Concerning the two light forms tested, "Broadband polychromatic PBM (non-thermal photobiomodulation) showed no advantage over the red-light-only spectrum."

Wound Healing

Given the reported ability of light-emitting diodes (LEDs) to send light deep into body tissues of the body, at wavelengths in a higher range (600-1000 nm), a meta-analysis of 68 studies on laser light and LED light was conducted to measure the effects on cutaneous wound healing, pain reduction, and tissue repair.

Results: "The biological effects promoted were reduction of inflammatory cells, increased proliferation of fibroblasts, stimulation of collagen synthesis, angiogenesis inducement and granulation tissue formation" (NIH, 2014). The study concludes that "phototherapy, either by LASER or LED, is an effective therapeutic modality to promote healing of skin wounds."

Rheumatoid Arthritis

Light therapy has been used as a short-term treatment to relieve arthritis pain and morning stiffness; it is "Now an FDA approved treatment: physicians use it to help patients suffering from chronic joint pain" (Red Light Clinic, 2022). Red light therapy is credited with collagen production stimulation, cellular rejuvenation, increased blood flow, and cartilage rebuilding, making it a "Favourable healing and preventative tool against the root causes of osteoarthritis, rheumatoid arthritis (RA), and various other inflammatory joint issues."

For verification, five studies were conducted among 130 randomly selected participants.

Results: LLLT (Low-Level Light Therapy) measurably reduced pain at a 95% confidence level, compared to placebo. It reduced morning stiffness duration by 27.5 minutes; and increased tip-to-palm flexibility by 1.3 cm. The study authors concluded that "LLLT could be considered for short-term treatment for relief of pain and morning stiffness for RA patients, particularly since it has few side effects."

Depression

Based on numerous studies, "Continual exposure to red light therapy has proven beneficial for individuals suffering from depression or fatigue," Red Light Clinic reports. These positive effects are based on the ability of red light wavelengths to actually penetrate facial skin, triggering subcutaneous neurons to increase the production of mood-elevating neurotransmitters.

Results. Patients who were fatigued, mildly depressed, or are susceptible to seasonal affective disorder have reported being happier, more energised, and more positive after being exposed to one-hour and two-hour light therapy. Given the potential of light therapy to provide a non-drug, rapidly acting treatment for a serious disorder like depression, further studies are being recommended.

Phototherapy at Different Wavelengths

Red Light at 600 nm to 650 nm

RLT at these low to midrange red light wavelengths is generally used as part of skin care regimens to improve skin health overall by smoothing fine lines and wrinkles, and softening rough spots, to achieve a better complexion:

- These effects are achieved by stimulating the production of collagen in the skin cells. These wavelengths "Significantly improved skin's firmness, thickness, and appearance," reports Red Light Clinic (2019), adding that these wavelengths have been used "To treat cellulite, stretch marks, acne, and other skin conditions such as psoriasis and rosacea."

- Furthermore, red light therapy at 600 nm to 650 nm wavelengths does more than improve the skin; it has been found in studies to make a person more focused and able to concentrate. "There's evidence it can increase alertness and performance—night shift workers exposed to 630 nm red light were more awake and did better in daily tasks than the control group."

Red Light at 650 nm to 700 nm

At this upper end of the visible red light wavelength spectrum, clinical trials found evidence of improved cell repair, resulting in a reduction of inflammation and encouragement of healing of wounds. The additional results of the application of this wavelength range include:

- Encouragement of hair growth because at 655 nm, red light can stimulate hair follicles that are in the dormant, or resting catagen phase, and return the follicles to the anagen, or growth phase. Hair loss like male pattern baldness, thinning and other types of alopecia can be mitigated.

- Improving sleep quality and duration. A study confirmed that red light with wavelengths near 658 nm helped those suffering from insomnia to fall asleep and stay asleep.

- More serious forms of skincare were recorded in a clinical trial conducted with burn victims. The RLT treatment at 670 nm smoothed and reduced scars and encouraged skin repair, as well as reduced pain.

Visible Red Light vs. Infrared Light Therapy

As you'll recall from our discussion of the spectrum, visible red light's wavelength ends at 700 nm, and that is where infrared light begins, extending to about 1,200 nm. You've probably seen or used IR lights to provide warming heat, but are there more therapeutic benefits?

Non-Visible IR light has been found to use its longer wavelengths therapeutically, providing these benefits, which confirm its penetrating power:

- Reducing pain: At wavelengths around 900 nm, IR therapy lowered pain and discomfort associated with tendonitis and joint issues, from strains to arthritis.

- "Help with some of the unpleasant side-effects of cancer treatment, such as oral mucositis and neuropathy" (Red Light Therapy, 2019).

- IR therapy encourages nerve repair and neural regeneration.

LED Phototherapy

LED light therapy is transmitted by light-emitting diodes, or LEDs, which you may be familiar with as ultra-intensive light bulbs, which emit intensive white light in a wide range of lighting applications, even security lights. They use less electricity and are brighter and longer lived than incandescent bulbs.

How LEDs work:

- Technically speaking, "A light-emitting diode is a semiconductor device that emits light when an electric current flows through it. When current passes through an LED, the electrons recombine with holes (created by the absence of electrons), emitting light in the process," explains *Byju's* (2022).

- In simplest terms, when an electric current is passed through an LED, "Energy is released in the form of photons. We call this phenomenon electroluminescence."

- The colours that are emitted are determined by chemicals used in the composition of the LED semiconducting material. Two primary materials are used for colours in LEDs: Aluminium gallium indium phosphide alloys produce yellow, orange, and red light; indium gallium nitride alloys produce green, blue, and white light.

For therapeutic applications, LED light is applied at various wavelengths that represent a range of visible colours (not just red), which penetrate the skin at different depths:

- Blue LED light is high frequency, very short wavelength light that affects the outermost layers of the skin. Blue light therapy is used to treat acne by destroying bacteria-causing bacteria; it also treats sun damage, and certain forms of skin cancer (squamous cell, basal cell).

- Yellow LED light therapy operates within wavelengths from 570 nm to 620 nm and has a relatively shallow level of penetration. It is claimed to help resolve skin redness, including rosacea and spider veins. It stimulates "Circulation and the production of red blood cells, which play a vital role in skin healing and skin cell rejuvenation."

- Red light travels even more deeply into your skin, and near-infrared light, beginning at the 700 nm limit of visible red light, penetrates deepest, to reduce inflammation and stimulates the production of collagen, the protein responsible for helping ageing skin become younger-looking skin.

Up next: Many benefits are claimed for RLT, but as we've indicated, the substantiating facts are only partially validated, and the therapeutic value of RLT has not yet been evaluated in depth; that's what we'll cover in the following chapter.

Julia E. Chatwin

Chapter 3 - Unveiling the Benefits of Red Light Therapy

"Science is simply common sense at its best." — *Thomas Huxley*[4]

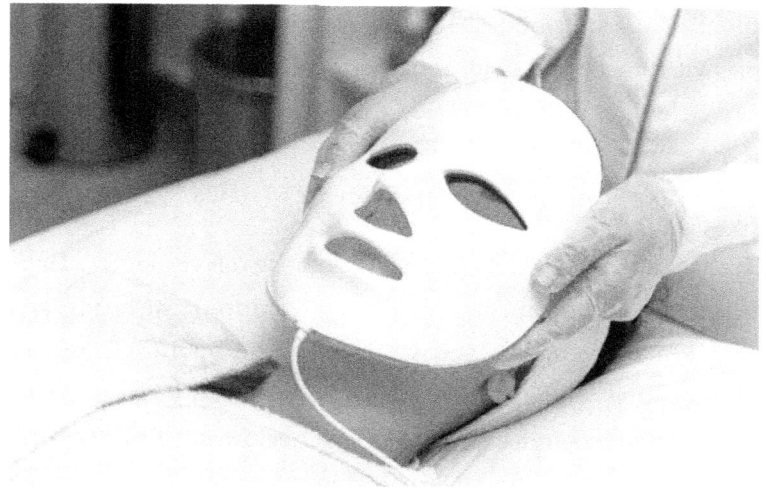

One thing is for sure—RLT has attracted considerable attention in recent years for its potential therapeutic benefits. As you turn the pages of this chapter, we will examine the various purported benefits it has to offer. But before we embark on this exploration, it is important to clarify the use of the term "purported". By no means do I intend to imply that these benefits are unproven, or mere claims. Instead, the term "purported" is used to acknowledge that our understanding of red light therapy is continually evolving, and new scientific research is constantly emerging to shed light on its efficacy.

---

[4] English biologist and anthropologist

To be clear, in this book, the approach is grounded in science. We will provide a balanced view of the benefits of red light therapy by examining the current body of scientific evidence, including peer-reviewed studies and clinical trials. This rigorous approach will allow us to present a comprehensive and unbiased analysis of the therapy's potential advantages and effectiveness. As we explore the various benefits together, I invite you to approach the topic with an open mind and a critical eye. By considering the scientific evidence, you will be better equipped to understand the true potential of red light therapy and make informed decisions about its application in your own life or practice.

RLT has gained traction due to its non-invasive nature, lack of side effects, and promising results in a multitude of health areas. From skin rejuvenation and wound healing to muscle recovery and cognitive enhancement, red light therapy is poised to revolutionise the landscape of modern healthcare. In this chapter, we will methodically explore the different domains where red light therapy has shown potential benefits. We will discuss the underlying mechanisms at play, review scientific evidence supporting its effectiveness, and provide insights into practical applications of this remarkable technology.

Join me on this enlightening journey as we shine a light on the myriad benefits of red light therapy, opening up a world of possibilities for improved health, wellness, and quality of life.

Being Able to Make an Informed Decision

One of the most important objectives of this book is to identify and elaborate upon the validated and confirmed benefits of using red light therapy and other forms of phototherapy. It will also indicate the claims of benefits that have not yet been proven.

The Scientific Method

To begin, it's important to understand the discipline known as the Scientific Method, which establishes the parameters of how to separate fact from what is unproven. You may recall earlier mention that a claim or hypothesis that is not proven and verified is not necessarily untrue or unprovable; in time, it might be validated, but for now, it cannot be accepted as truth or fact.

But what qualifies as proven? At one extreme, a randomised, double-blind, placebo-controlled large-scale study produces findings that are up to 99% significant in their accuracy and can be projected to a larger population. The recent Covid-19 vaccine clinical trials conducted by Pfizer, Moderna, Johnson & Johnson, AstraZeneca, and other major laboratories, used matched samples of 10,000 participants (one sample group received the real vaccine; the other sample group received an inactive placebo). This is an example of research findings that can be trusted.

- Matched samples (or matched pairs) mean all the participants were chosen at random, and the sample groups were matched in age, gender, geographic location, physical condition, and other factors.

- Double-blind means neither the participant nor the researcher recording the results knows whether the participant received the drug or the placebo.

Anecdotal. At the other extreme of what is proven or statistically validated is what is known as anecdotal claims; something that is repeated in publications, and between people by word of mouth, and is treated as fact, even though it has not been clinically or scientifically tested. Examples of this phenomenon abound:

- **Claim:** Drinking coffee stunts children's growth and development.
- **Reality check:** While excessive caffeine intake can have negative effects, moderate caffeine consumption is considered safe for children and there is no evidence to suggest that coffee can stunt childhood development.
- **Claim:** Breakfast is the most important meal of the day.
- **Reality check:** This may have had relevance when we were working in agriculture, but dietary studies show we do better with our caloric intake spread across the day.
- **Claim:** Eating before bed makes you overweight
- **Reality check:** Some studies have suggested that eating before bed can actually be beneficial for weight management. One study published in the British Journal of Nutrition found that eating a high-protein snack before bed helped to increase muscle mass and improve metabolic health in overweight and obese adults.
- **Claim:** You need to drink 8 cups of water a day.
- **Reality check:** We get frequent reminders to avoid dehydration, but unless you're hiking across a desert, or see that your urine is dark, you can ratchet back to 5 or 6 cups safely. I should add I am a big fan of staying hydrated and I personally drink **at least** 8 cups a day. But is serves as an example here!

- **Claim:** Senior men and women must take a daily multivitamin to protect their health and longevity.
- **Reality check:** "There is little scientific proof that multivitamins or special 'senior' vitamin formulas help you live longer, feel better, or avoid disease. Spending money on fresh fruits and vegetables is a wiser and healthier investment" (*Harvard Health,* 2016).

Observational. Another type of questionable claim is when it's based on limited or observational evidence. For example, when 10 or 20 people experience a benefit; the results may justify conducting more studies to learn more, but should not be accepted until the validation is completed.

Non-human studies. Another type of limited evidence is when positive laboratory results of a new drug trial are based on tests with mice or other non-human subjects. Given previous histories of animal studies leading to life-saving medications, lab animal tests, when positive, can give a green light to proceed to human trials, but until those human studies are completed under the scientific security and disciplines, we've been discussing, the findings are encouraging, but definitely not yet validated.

Bias or influence is another cause of claims that aren't trustable. Market researchers who understand statistics and what makes up the reliability of study findings are frustrated when focus groups are used to make important decisions. Ten people in a room discussing a new product do not represent a national population (or any population), and worse, the opinions participants express during the focus groups are heavily biassed by what others have said, and by what the group moderator may have implied while leading the discussion.

We can sum up this review of the need to question the benefits of red light therapy, and all claimed medical results, by adopting a "healthy scepticism" until you know for sure that scientific methods have been followed, and the results have been validated. With all this understood, we can now get serious about looking into RLT's effects and effectiveness.

"Red light therapy (RLT) is a treatment that *may help* skin, muscle tissue, and other parts of your body heal," declares *WebMD* (2019). Just as in an earlier quote from Cleveland Clinic, this description contains an important conditional phrase. It's a big leap from *"may help"* to *"will help."* We have some sorting out to do that will separate the proven from the unproven.

Let's take it one benefit at a time, keeping in mind that one RLT treatment that is confirmed to be effective in treating one symptom or problem does not mean it will also be effective in solving or relieving a different problem or disorder; conversely, it's worth repeating that a treatment or therapy's failure to perform as promised should not negate its potential to be effective in other areas.

How to evaluate the following information about RLT benefits:

- In addition to the studies that are cited to validate the effectiveness of the benefits, some of the findings and successes with RLT are recommended by medical professionals, including board-certified dermatologists for skin and hair treatment.

- These are trustworthy authorities, whose recommendations are based on their review of clinical trials and other studies, and often combined with their own professional experiences in treating patients.

Benefits to the Skin

This will be the largest category of RLT applications for us to cover because there are many skin-related problems that are effectively treatable by RLT. The skin deserves our fullest attention because it is the body's first line of defence against potential invading pathogens. It provides an almost impenetrable shield, and an acidic barrier that deters bacteria and viruses.

In addition, "A new Yale study shows that the epidermis, the outermost layer of skin, consists of an army of immune cells that station themselves at regular intervals across the skin's vast expanse to resist infection" (*Yale News*, 2019).

But despite these protections, our skin has many vulnerabilities. These range from diseases and injuries, to disturbances in a person's appearance, which can deeply affect their self-esteem:

- The skin is actually an organ; the largest in our bodies and is subject to a host of injuries and insults, from rashes, acne, hyperpigmentation, rosacea, bug bites and inflammation, to bacterial and fungal infections, and skin cancer.

- Skin may carry scars from burns, cuts, and other wounds, residual marks from previous infections and other trauma, and may display stretch marks resulting from skin expansions and contractions caused by pregnancy or weight changes.

- And to the consternation of people as they age, skin tends to develop fine lines and wrinkles. It can also can become tissue thin; the slightest scratch can cause a deep gash. Ageing of the skin is a natural process and causes no discomfort, at least physically, but mentally it can be a frustrating signal of ageing, displayed for all to see on the face and hands. In addition to cellular causes, sun damage is a primary cause of premature wrinkles, along with many other skin problems.

- Unlike all of the interior parts of our body, the skin is what we, and others see, and react to. The $164 billion global skincare industry (*Statista* 2022) has grown steadily to meet the increasing demand for skin treatments with creams, gels, lotions, and medications taken both topically and orally; the question now is whether red light therapy can provide superior benefits and become a dermatologically accepted skin care alternative.

How RLT Works

What are the skin conditions that RLT is used to treat, and how effective are they?

"Red light therapy (RLT) involves exposing the skin to safe wavelengths of light in order to address several skin concerns, including signs of ageing, stretch marks, scars, hyperpigmentation, and acne," according to board-certified cosmetic dermatologist Dr. Dendy Engelman, at the Shafer Clinic for skin care in New York City (*Women's Health,* (2022):

- "Low wavelength red light produces a biochemical effect in cells," which enables the mitochondria in the cells to generate more energy to help cells to "work more efficiently to rejuvenate and repair damage."

- "Red light can penetrate up to five millimetres into the skin without causing any thermal damage," notes another board-certified dermatologist, Dr. Jessie Cheung, who identifies this advantage of RLT skin care treatments: "It can be effective without being invasive."

- RLT is most frequently administered professionally with a panel of LEDs at an aesthetician or dermatologist's practice, but there are also at-home treatment options, including RLT wands, and face masks (home use of RLT-emitting devices is covered in a later chapter).

Dr. Engleman highlights (no pun intended) the particular benefits of RLT compared to other types of light therapy. "This technology is so great because it is completely painless and doesn't cause damage to the skin or downtime, like some other light therapies (at different wavelengths and colours) can do." (Although there are situations when multiple colour lights are used, as you'll read in a moment in the section about acne.)

A key advantage of RLT is its stimulation and encouragement of skin regeneration, or new cellular growth, in contrast to other therapies that "Stimulate tissue repair by causing controlled damage to the outermost layer of the skin," Dr. Engleman adds, citing RLT's important benefits of reducing scars, wrinkles, and acne; safely and effectively, as explained in the following.

Treating Acne

Acne, a common yet often misunderstood skin condition, can have profound effects on both physical and emotional well-being. Affecting millions of people worldwide, acne is characterised by the appearance of pimples, blackheads, whiteheads, and even cysts, which can lead to scarring and discolouration if not properly treated. Beyond the visible symptoms, the psychological impact of acne should not be underestimated. Individuals suffering from this condition may experience social anxiety, low self-esteem, and even depression, which can significantly impair their daily functioning and quality of life. As such, it is crucial to recognise the serious nature of acne and strive to find effective solutions that address both the physical manifestations and the emotional challenges it presents.

Red light is more effective than other wavelengths in penetrating deeply into the skin, where it can stop the formation of pimples at "the source by targeting the sebaceous glands' production of sebum, according to a 2015 study in the *Indian Dermatology Online Journal*." RLT stimulates the production of collagen to "improve the skin's healing abilities, making it great for treating acne," says Dr. Engelman.

- Yet there are situations when red light can be coupled with blue light for more effective results. As explained by Dr.

Dhaval Bhanusali, founder of Skin Medicinals, and a board-certified, New York City-based dermatologist, some research findings suggest "Red light should be coupled with blue light for a synergistic effect, as blue light is said to target the bacteria that can cause acne and the red light may actually be more effective at treating residual redness" (*Women's Health,* (2022).

Sun Damage

Whether it's from casual sun exposure over the years, or efforts to obtain a tan, our skin suffers damage from the sun. The results include spots and dark areas, premature wrinkles, the onset of squamous cell and basal cell carcinomas, and the more dangerous metastatic melanomas.

Can light therapy reverse years of accumulated sun damage?

- There is ample evidence that "RLT helps heal sun damage by reducing inflammation and increasing collagen and elastin production to boost the skin's repair processes," according to Dr. Engelman.

Important: RLT may slow or stop the progression of squamous and basal cell pre-carcinomas, but a dermatologist's intervention is strongly advised for an evaluation and possible biopsy and is mandatory for cases of melanoma, which can be fatal if untreated.

Healing Wounds and Scars

"The healing benefits come from red light wavelength's ability to reduce inflammation," says Dr. Nazanin Saedi, M.D., clinical associate professor at Thomas Jefferson University, and a board-certified dermatologist in Philadelphia. Because red light stimulates the mitochondria in your skin cells to produce ATP, the source of cellular energy, this effect can lead to new cells turning over, and tissues repairing faster. A series of studies on the effects of LLLT to stimulate, heal, and restore skin (National Institutes of Health, 2014) concluded that "Scars and burns are particularly responsive to red light therapy."

According to Dr. Saedi, reducing inflammation may be the most important benefit of red light therapy. Furthermore, Dr. Cheung explains that "RLT can boost production of antioxidants and reduce oxidative stress, which can also reduce inflammation."

- Dr. Engelman adds that "Red light is effective at reducing inflammation because it triggers the formation of blood vessels and increases production of collagen and fibroblasts," since these actions can lower inflammation.

Anti-Ageing and Wrinkles

To understand the potential of RLT to help reduce fine lines and wrinkles, you need to know about collagen:

- Collagen is a structural protein; the most abundant in our bodies. Structural proteins form the framework of our tissues and cells. Among the 28 known types of collagen, type I collagen accounts for about 90% of the collagen in our body.

- Being a protein, collagen is built up from amino acids: proline, hydroxyproline, and glycine. "These amino acids form three strands, which make up the triple-helix structure characteristic of collagen" (*Healthline,* 2022).

Here's where it gets interesting: Collagen provides structural support to our skin, connective tissues, tendons, cartilage, and bones, and is active in cellular processes. To be clear, our skin depends on collagen to keep its shape, which is why collagen has been called "the skin's fountain of youth."

Unfortunately, our levels of collagen in the skin decrease with age, and with the damage caused by the sun, air pollution, smoking, and other causes of dryness (even air conditioning), collagen production is further reduced. The result is dry, inelastic, sagging skin, often appearing well before the senior years arrive.

The positive effects of RLT in helping to reduce fine lines and wrinkles depend on its ability to stimulate collagen; this is where RLT has been tested and proven to play an important role in reversing the ageing effects:

- "By stimulating collagen and elastin production, red light therapy helps reduce fine lines and wrinkles, giving skin a more youthful appearance," Dr. Engelman concludes. The red light wavelength penetrates to reach and enter the cells and their mitochondrial energy factories to deliver additional energy, without causing damage to mitochondria or DNA.

Melasma: Treat or Make Worse?

What is it? "Melasma is a pigmentation disorder of the skin mostly affecting women, especially those with darker skin," according to

Harvard Health Publishing (2022). This condition is typically seen on the face, as patches with irregular borders and dark spots. Melasma is not harmful physically, but studies cited by the National Institutes of Health have shown that the condition "Can lead to psychological problems and poorer quality of life due to the changes it causes in a person's appearance."

- The importance of protecting people from facial appearance insecurities cannot be underestimated. As a result, people subject to this condition can become anxious and open to trying alternative treatments.

While at first, Melasma seems to be a rare disorder, affecting just 1% of the general population, that can rise to 50% among those in higher-risk groups, including people with darker skin. Melasma is called the "mask of pregnancy" because of pregnancy-induced hormonal changes; it is also associated with birth control pills, another hormonal source of the excessive skin pigment production characteristic of melasma. Exposure to the sun also plays a significant role in the development of melasma.

Melasma is **not fully preventable** among those who are likely to develop it due to their hormones, skin colour and type, and genetic profile. Given their high level of sensitivity to sunlight, they are advised to avoid direct sun exposure, especially during peak hours, to diligently apply high-SPF sunscreens, and not to take hormonal medications, if possible, to help protect against melasma flares and their recurrence.

The Potential of Red Light Therapy

While there is **no cure yet** available, red light therapy has built a reputation for being an effective treatment to reduce the appearance of Melasma's dark spots. *Harvard Health Publishing* explains: "Laser therapies can destroy pigment cells in skin and therefore lighten the dark spots in melasma." But there is a caution that, "as with any other treatment option for melasma, there is considerable risk of relapse post-treatment".

There are conflicting concerns, however, that red light and other phototherapy may cause the spots of melasma to form. Based on what is known so far, red light appears to be safe, as long as the devices being used are verified UV wavelength-free.

The Cleveland Clinic (2022) warns those susceptible to melasma to avoid "LED light from your television, laptop, cell phone, and tablet."

Does this imply that any light therapy is to be avoided? Kiayan Medical (2021) says light therapy can be beneficial, and advocates, "There is a non-invasive and non-pharmacological approach, and it uses the power of light," referring, of course, to RLT:

- Red light therapy's wavelengths can penetrate the skin, "stimulating the production of adenosine triphosphate (ATP) within the mitochondria" (as we've explained, ATP is the "powerhouse of the cells, responsible for storing and transferring energy in the body's cells").

- Thus, damaged and old cells can be repaired, and new cells can be created. "As a result, the body can naturally heal itself, improve the texture and appearance of the skin, and increase collagen production," explains Kiayan Medical, citing studies to research the positive effects of red light therapy in treating melasma.

The studies referred to are extensive and show various responses to different types of light transmission and therapy, including augmentation to topical chemical applications that were not effective on their own. The source reporting these findings, the *International Journal of Women's Dermatology* (2017), concludes:

"Laser and light therapy for the treatment of melasma is best suited for patients with refractory melasma who failed with topical treatment or a series of chemical peels."

- Light and laser therapy is an alternative approach to treat patients with recalcitrant melasma. As advancements in laser and LED device technologies evolve the treatments will continue to improve.

See a Dermatologist

With the diversity of light wavelength therapy approaches that are available; the different skin conditions to be treated; and the variety of methods of how to treat each case; it is strongly recommended that those who need to treat melasma with light therapy only do so under the supervision of a trained medical authority, preferably a dermatologist.

It is important to realise that each person's skin is unique and will react to treatments, topical lotions and medications, and phototherapy in a unique manner. Curing melasma is important, but taking care not to damage your skin is far more important.

Blood Pressure Benefits

High blood pressure, also known as hypertension, is a leading risk factor for cardiovascular disease, which remains the leading cause of death globally. Managing blood pressure levels is therefore an essential component of maintaining heart health. Fortunately, a growing body of evidence suggests that infrared light therapy may be a safe and effective non-pharmacological intervention for reducing blood pressure levels. Several clinical studies have shown that regular infrared light therapy sessions can lead to a significant reduction in both systolic and diastolic blood pressure. For example, a 2018 study published in the Journal of Clinical Hypertension found that six weeks of infrared light therapy sessions led to a significant reduction in both systolic and diastolic blood pressure in hypertensive patients.

Similarly, a 2016 study published in the journal Photomedicine and Laser Surgery found that 12 weeks of infrared light therapy sessions led to a significant reduction in both systolic and diastolic blood pressure in patients with prehypertension. In both studies, the reductions in blood pressure were maintained even after the treatment period, suggesting that infrared light therapy may have a lasting effect on blood pressure levels.

The exact mechanisms by which infrared light therapy reduces blood pressure levels are not fully understood. However, it is thought that the therapy works, by again enhancing nitric oxide production. The Nitric oxide helps to dilate blood vessels and increase blood flow, which can help to reduce blood pressure levels. We have learnt (from the previous chapter) how RLT increases nitric oxide production in the skin, which may translate to increased production in the blood vessels and ultimately lead to a reduction in blood pressure.

Another potential mechanism by which infrared light therapy reduces blood pressure levels is through its ability to reduce inflammation. Chronic inflammation is a known contributor to hypertension, and several studies have shown that infrared light therapy can reduce inflammation in various tissues throughout the body.

Benefits to the Hair and Scalp

From a dermatological perspective, hair and scalp are within the skincare category, but for clarity, are reviewed here separately because of their unique characteristics. Like the skin, the hair is visible to all. Its condition can be, on one hand, a source of pride. On the other hand, a source of discomfort, or even self-conscious embarrassment:

- Hair loss, or alopecia, is an especially concerning hair and scalp condition, and can be experienced by women as well as men. While androgenic alopecia, or male pattern baldness, characterised by a gradually receding hairline and a bald spot on top, is limited to men; both genders can experience alopecia areata, or patchy hair loss, and other forms of loss that increasingly reveal the scalp.

- There is also chemotherapy-induced hair loss, which occurs during treatment for cancer. However, this often resolves after treatment is concluded.

- Some hair loss and scalp disorders, like itchiness and scabs forming, can result from infections, or illness, and are caused by vitamin deficiencies, and hormone imbalances (which we'll cover separately, next). Male pattern baldness is generally an inherited condition; topical and oral treatments (Minoxidil and Propecia) have had some success in slowing or even reversing the condition.

Your hair grows from tiny hair follicles in the scalp, and each hair shaft is in one of three lifecycle phases:

- **Phase 1:** Anagen phase is when hair is healthy and growing and is not easily pulled out (it actually hurts if pulled!). In a healthy, normal scalp, most hair is in the anagen phase.
- **Phase 2:** Catagen phase is when hair is no longer growing, but in a resting stage; in catagen, hair is not easily pulled out, and depending on conditions, may be reactivated to the anagen phase, or may descend to the third phase.
- **Phase 3:** Telogen is the final lifecycle phase when hair can no longer grow and falls or pulls out easily. Hair that you find on the hairbrush or in the sink is telogen phase hair. Once it enters telogen, hair shafts cannot be revived.

Can phototherapy intervene and prevent hair loss by reviving catagen phase hair to the growth phase anagen phase? Can RLT resolve scalp infections and deficiencies to increase the percentage of healthy growing hair to exceed the percentage of hair that is falling out?

While red light therapy may not be a "Magic bullet for restoring hair to its original state, studies have shown that red light waves can stimulate hair follicles into production." (*Women's Health*, 2022). Dr. Bhanusali is uncertain about the precise mechanism behind these positive results but thinks it could be a "Function of RLT's anti-inflammatory properties, the increase in blood flow it creates, or the spike in collagen production it can cause."

Dr. Bhanusali has achieved success treating hair loss in his own practice, by using a red light laser after "PRP (platelet-rich plasma) hair rejuvenation sessions" to treat various forms of alopecia. "In the office, we do them weekly for hair loss as needed (and same for rejuvenation) for about four to six sessions," he reports.

Benefits to Balance Hormones

Red light therapy is believed to help maintain optimal hormone levels by stabilising circadian rhythms to help you sleep better, energising cells by increasing energy production (via ATP) in the mitochondria and helping balance the intestinal microbiome, which communicates with the brain. These processes are thought to improve hormone production, but many of these claims are not as well substantiated as those relating to skin care.

Perhaps one of the most important applications of RLT is for the treatment of the thyroid gland, where many hormones are produced. The National Center for Biotechnology Information (2018) defines the thyroid as a vital hormone gland that plays a "Major role in the metabolism, growth, and development of the human body." The thyroid helps to "Regulate many body functions by constantly releasing a steady amount of thyroid hormones into the bloodstream." The thyroid gland produces additional hormones on an as-needed basis.

The butterfly-shaped thyroid gland is positioned at the front of the neck, beneath the voice box. It consists of two side lobes around the windpipe, or trachea, which make the gland easily accessible to red light therapy.

But what can RLT do to affect the thyroid's hormone production? *Higher Dose* (2022) states that "Today, the medical community and health care practitioners have also included red light therapy in their pro-thyroid health arsenal for auto-immune disorders, including certain thyroid conditions."

By energising the mitochondria within the organ, it "enables the thyroid cells to function optimally, adjusting your hormonal supply based on your body's needs."

- "It helps reduce medication time in Hashimoto thyroiditis (hypothyroidism)," as confirmed by Dr. D.B. Höfling of Brazil's University of Sao Paulo Medical School, who led a study on the effects of red light therapy on hypothyroidism. He "Discovered that close to 50% of those who participated in the experiment were able to entirely stop taking medication during the nine months of follow-up."

- "It protects your thyroid against natural killer cells," which can overreact and cause autoimmune damage to the thyroid's cells. "Research shows that red light therapy can reduce the presence of thyroid antibodies and prevent auto-immune disorders from interfering with your thyroid's normal processes."

Benefits that Relieve Pain

Traditional pain-killing medications work by blocking the perception of pain, while red light therapy works at the cellular level to promote mitochondrial and cellular health by "Reducing inflammation, which then reduces pain signals at the source."

Red and near-infrared light therapy activate the production of stem cells to support the healing process. "Stem cells are non-specialised cells that are present in an inactive state throughout the body," When there is a need for stem cells, for example, as a result of injuries, infections, or damage to any of the body's trillions of cells, embryonic stem cells travel in the bloodstream to the affected area, where "they develop into any cell that's needed" for immediate repairs.

Pain is a normal and natural response that your body uses to warn you to stop a specific behaviour or action that may be harmful.

- Acute pain occurs when you touch a hot stove or step on something sharp, and in a fraction of a second, the signal travels through the spinal cord to the brain where it is processed, and a pain message is signalled back to the area of trauma, which then initiates a response. For example, pulling your hand off the stove before you're even aware of the problem. If there's no serious damage, the pain will subside on its own.

- Chronic pain is when pain persists long after the needed reaction occurs, during the healing process, and even longer, becoming a chronic form of pain. Chronic or intermittently continuing pain may be relieved by red light therapy.

- Neuropathic pain is caused by disturbances to the nervous system from diseases and injuries and may be continuous or intermittent. Sources of pain can be inflammation, spinal disc compression (sciatica), MS, Parkinson's, carpal tunnel, shingles, and chemotherapy. The degree to which RLT's deep penetration can reach and calm the neurons responsible for the pain will determine how effective it can be.

Benefits that Relieve Arthritis and Tendonitis

The Centers for Disease Control and Prevention (CDC), reports that "54 million Americans suffer from arthritis, and 60 percent are under the age of 65" (*Platinum Therapy Lights*, 2021). These include about 8 million people who find it challenging, and in some cases, impossible to work because of their condition. While osteoarthritis (cartilage degradation in joints) and rheumatoid arthritis (autoimmune caused) respond to some medications, many patients are receptive to non-drug, non-invasive alternatives.

Some early research reported by the *British Journal of Sports Medicine* (2006), a "randomised, placebo-controlled trial of low-level laser therapy for activated Achilles tendinitis" and joint discomfort with microdialysis measurement demonstrated that red light therapy can potentially reduce the discomfort and pain associated with osteoarthritis and rheumatoid arthritis.

This and later studies have found that the effectiveness of these treatments is credited to RLT's anti-inflammatory properties. "By increasing blood circulation and stimulating the body's healing processes, RLT helps reduce pain from tendonitis and arthritis," says Dr. Engelman. These studies (*Platinum Therapy Lights*, 2021) corroborate the findings:

- A team of Brazilian researchers conducted a study in 2019 that "Found that exposure to red and near-infrared light is an effective way to stimulate collagen production in the joints." The research found that red light therapy encouraged "Cartilage recovery and reduced the progression of cartilage degradation, which suggests a potential role for red light in treating chronic osteoarthritis."

- A 2017 study in Saudi Arabia also found that red light therapy "Helps increase the regeneration and thickness of cartilage and reduce osteoarthritis pain." Knee osteoarthritis patients received low-level laser therapy three days per week over a four-week test and were also tested eight weeks after the conclusion of the treatment. "Researchers found significant differences in pain relief and improved cartilage thickness."

- Red light therapy effectively treated tears in the meniscus, the cartilage in the front part of the knee joint, in a 2013 clinical trial. "Four weeks after receiving red light therapy, the treatment group reported a statistically significant decrease of symptoms compared to the placebo group." The study concluded that light therapy is a viable alternative "For patients with meniscal tears who do not wish to undergo surgery."

Benefits to Increase Energy

There is clinically derived evidence that photobiomodulation, including red light therapy, can increase energy and athletic performance.

According to the NIH's National Centre for Biotechnology Information (2017):

- "The rationale for using photobiomodulation on muscles relies on the well-known stimulation of mitochondrial activity that occurs after red or near-infrared photons delivered to the tissue have been absorbed by cytochrome c oxidase."

- You will recall from the previous chapter that muscles depend on adenosine triphosphate (ATP), the biological source of energy required for muscle movement. Thus, increased ATP levels are a recognised hypothesis to explain the impressive effects that red light therapy seems to exert on muscle tissue.

- In addition, there are other mechanisms of action to explain the effects of red light therapy on muscle cells and tissues, and the resultant improvement in sports performance.

Benefits that Improve Sexual Function

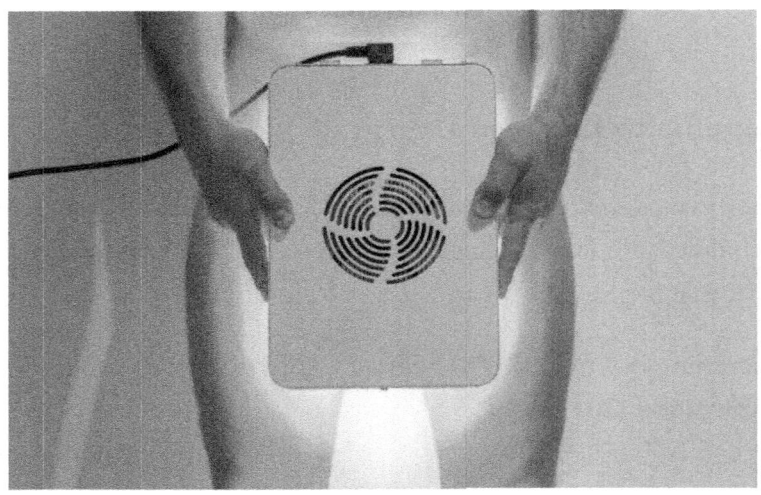

In addition to the explanation of mitochondrial activities influenced by light therapy in the preceding section on energy, you will recall in the last chapter our reporting that red light therapy's waves can penetrate the skin to reach and energise the mitochondria in our cells.

"It also causes an increase in nitric oxide (NO), which dilates blood vessels and helps improve blood flow, according to a 2017 article published in AIMS Biophysics," which is cited by sexuality editor Kay Johnson in the health publication *Giddy* (2022).

Do dilated blood vessels and improved circulation—which leads to increased energy—also lead to improved sexual function? There is speculation that RLT may prevent erectile dysfunction and vaginal dryness. "However, there has been little research in this area, and most of the benefits for women's health are speculative," Ms. Johnson says.

Benefits to Control Dementia

Dementia describes a loss of the normal ability to think, as well as diminished memory, logical reasoning, attentiveness, and other mental faculties. Dementia is diagnosed when these changes and conditions regularly interfere with occupational or social functioning.

Dementia, also called a major neurocognitive disorder, has many causes but happens when "Parts of your brain used for learning, memory, decision making, and language are diseased," explains *WebMD* (2022). Dementia isn't so much a disease but is a "group of symptoms caused by other conditions."

Dementia affects between 5% to 8% of adults who are over age 65; Alzheimer's disease is the most common cause. Dementia symptoms may improve with treatment, including red light therapy, "But many of the diseases that cause dementia aren't curable," notably Alzheimer's, which affects at least 60% of dementia cases.

Unfortunately, there is little scientific evidence to support claims made by advertisers of RLT equipment that red light therapy has positive effects on dementia. The British Alzheimer's Society (2022) sums up the state of the research:

- "More evidence is needed before we can recommend using light therapy to help treat dementia and its symptoms."

- Several research studies have been conducted with light therapy as a treatment for dementia. "However, a greater number of clinical studies, with more participants, is needed before we can come to any conclusions."

The British Alzheimer's Society goes on to cite very limited research using bright light (white, not red) as showing promise for improving sleep patterns by regulating circadian rhythm, and also a helmet-applied application using near-infrared light, supposedly for the light to reach the brain—but there is no evidence this has any effect on dementia.

Side effects; causes or cures. Given concerns about skin damage from the sun, we can question whether red light therapy's penetration of the layers of the skin poses health and safety risks. We address the possibility of RLT's side effects next.

Chapter 4 - Shedding Light on Safety Concerns

"The science of today is the technology of tomorrow." — Edward Teller[5]

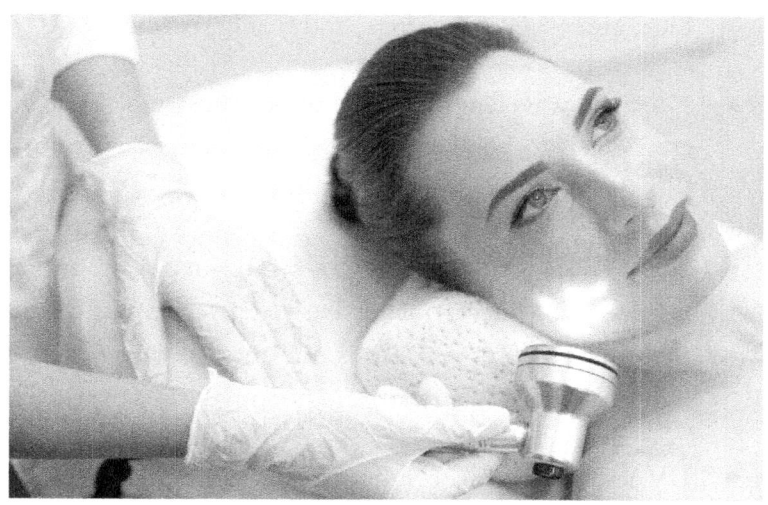

We Know About the Risks of UV, but What About Red Light Therapy?

Is it safe? This is a question we all ask when the benefits and applications of red light therapy—or any light therapy—are considered. A few generations ago, light, especially sunlight, was considered beneficial, and there were no risks, except for sunburn.

---

[5] Hungarian-American theoretical physicist

But not today. Now we are educated about the downsides of too much exposure to the wrong kinds of light, especially the sun's ultraviolet UVA and UVB wavelengths:

- UV resides on the wavelength spectrum just shorter than visible light; before progressively longer violet, indigo, blue, green, yellow, orange, and finally red.

- Note the wavelength separation between violet and red; consider it to be like a barrier that protects us from the threats that UV light poses.

- The threats of UV light go far beyond sunburn and include skin cancer, notably basal cell, squamous cell, and the much more dangerous melanoma, which can be metastatic (able to spread) and potentially life-threatening.

- UVA rays also cause sunburn and can damage the skin; UVB are the cause of premature wrinkles and other signs of ageing, including permanent dark spots and blemishes.

If you have been to see the dermatologist lately, you may have seen videos that warn about these risks and advocate the use of sunblock (okay, the doctor's office may be promoting the sale of sun protection products, but it's a beneficial intention). You may also see warnings about **tanning studios**; these are **to be avoided**, given solid data that confirms the increased risks of skin cancer and other skin damage from UV tanning beds.

Red Light Specifically

You've been reading, chapter by chapter, about red light therapy; here's some additional perspective. As we just covered, you know now about the dangers of sunlight and any other source of UVA and UVB light.

But what about red light, or near red light? You've read that red light's wavelengths can penetrate the skin; the outer layer called the epidermis and the inner dermis. This enables the stimulation of the energy-generating mitochondria in the subcutaneous layers, but at what cost? Is this penetration dangerous? Let's see:

- "Unlike ultraviolet rays from the sun which damage the DNA of skin cells, and can lead to serious problems, light emitted in this spectrum is perfectly safe," according to Dr. Susan Bard, a New York City board-certified dermatologist, quoted in *Healthline* (2019).

- But rest assured you don't have to worry about burning or tanning resulting from exposure to red light. The wavelengths of red and near-infrared ensure that the effects take place "Deep inside at the cellular level," *Healthline* counsels.

Red and near-red light therapy are generally considered safe, with few reported side effects. However, some possible side effects may include:

- Skin irritation: Some people may experience skin irritation, such as redness or itching, from prolonged exposure to red and near-red light.

- Headaches: In rare cases, people may experience headaches as a side effect of light therapy.

- Insomnia: Exposure to red and near-red light at night may disrupt sleep patterns and cause insomnia in some people.

- Hyperpigmentation: In rare cases, red and near-red light therapy may cause hyperpigmentation, or an increase in skin pigmentation.

- There's also a potential risk of damage to the eyes. Direct exposure to red and near-red light can cause damage to the retina, leading to potential vision problems. "Sit or stand a few inches away from a panel of special red lights for a few minutes and their wavelengths reportedly alter the way your cells produce energy and antioxidants." By improving the efficiency of the cell and their mitochondrial powerhouses, you may help to heal and repair skin, nerves, bones, ligaments, and tendons, while lowering pain. Proper eye protection may be necessary while undergoing red light therapy.

Red light therapy, and other types of phototherapies, are not new breakthrough discoveries but have been in use for over 50 years, although it's only in recent years that it has been more widely accepted by medical experts. Yet, the *extent* to which RLT is *accepted* ranges from enthusiastic to sceptical.

- Be careful when conducting an online search for RLT; you will see many highly positive reviews and ratings, but these are invariably from the retailers and distributors who are selling the RLT devices. Some may cite studies that are not trustable and fail to mention any risks.

- This book has been written based on the research findings, conclusions, and recommendations reported by reputable medical sources, like the Mayo Clinic, Harvard Health Publishing, the Cleveland Clinic, and news sources including *Healthline* and *WebMD*, and you should trust those same medical sources if you want to dig deeper (you can find all of the links to these sources at the end of the book).

LED lights that emit colours have existed since the 1960s, but more recently have been used in various forms of skin treatment, depending on the nature of their penetration. *Harvard Health Publishing* (2019) reminds us that "Different wavelengths of the visible light spectrum correspond to different colours of LED light and penetrate the skin to different depths." The biological effects they achieve, and the biological impact they have, are determined by the depth of their penetration.

Most studies come to the conclusion that, among the colours of the spectrum, **red light appears to pose no risks** while offering the benefits of being able to penetrate the skin and reach subcutaneous tissues and provide beneficial therapies, as discussed in the previous chapter. Near-infrared light, just adjacent to red on the spectrum with a slightly longer wavelength, is similarly considered safe and therapeutic:

- **Safety.** "For the most part, these LED light therapies (using red and blue light) appear to be relatively safe, at least in the short term," according to Dr. Elizabeth Buzney, an assistant dermatology professor at Harvard Medical School. (We'll get to blue light treatments later on.)

- On the subject of light therapy devices for home use, she states that "LED skin devices don't have a lot of power, so they're unlikely to burn your skin."

Protecting Your Eyes

On the scale of concerns about the safety of phototherapy, potential risks to the eyes certainly top the list. Our vision is precious, at every age, and it's normal to be careful not to do anything to cause eye damage. So, it's surprising that some people are trusting when exposing themselves to light therapy.

Our eyes are highly sensitive organs that receive light waves and focus them to the retina at the back of the eye, where the optic nerve transmits the information to the brain. The impulses are converted by the brain into visual images, and we see. Through countless generations, our eyes have adapted to perform these functions as long as there is visible light, but not too intense. It's a question of what wavelengths are entering your eyes, and at what intensity.

If you try to look directly at the sun when it's high in the sky on a clear day, the reflexes in your eyes make it very clear, very quickly, that this is dangerous. The intensity of the visible and near visible light (UV and IR) send signals from your brain, causing you to react for self-protection by forcing your eyes shut.

But the light used in phototherapy, at any visible or non-visible wavelength does not "warn you off" with intense pain; rather, you usually feel nothing. If some infrared light is emitted with other wavelengths, it may cause some warmth, and that is not dangerous as long as it's not too intense.

Similarly, red, blue, and white visible light are without risk as long as intensities are constrained and should cause no discomfort. But as you will need to know, should there be any UVA or UVB (or both) wavelengths, although you might not be aware of this, your eyes could still be damaged.

The message is clear: good quality, tested, and approved light-emitting devices are vital. If uncertain about the safety of a device, it's best not to use it, or at least take extra precautions to protect your eyes.

Precautions

This leads us to protecting our eyes during light therapy. The skin may be safe if the lights are used responsibly, but the most immediate potential risk from using colour therapy is eye damage. "It is important to shield your eyes from the light while using them," Harvard Medical School's Dr. Buzney advises.

For example, concerns over the potential risks of light therapy caused a nationwide product recall of one popular light therapy acne mask. The reason for this was due to a concern regarding potential damage to the eyes of patients with existing eye conditions. Or indeed, patients whose eyes have become light-sensitive due to ongoing medication use:

- "For a small subset of the population with certain underlying eye conditions, as well as for users taking medications which could enhance ocular photosensitivity, there is a theoretical risk of eye injury," the company explained in a statement (ABC 7 News, 2019).

- The mask was developed using two separate colour lights: To prevent acne breakouts, using "Blue light therapy to target acne-causing bacteria, and red light therapy to reduce inflammation."

- The company in question stated the recall was called "out of an abundance of caution," even though the mask was considered to be safe when used once per day as directed.

- The abundance of caution was due to the potential seriousness of causing eye damage, but in reality, the risks were few, with the company reporting that mask users' reactions included "Transient eye pain or irritation, tearing, blurry vision, seeing spots, or changes in colour vision" that were fully resolved, without lingering effects, shortly after discontinuing use of the mask.

- In total, the problems were rarely experienced, with "Complaints on about 0.02% of masks sold at the time of the recall." But this history underscores the high level of sensitivity people have when it comes to possibly damaging their eyes, and an underlying caution about using light waves on their faces.

Pregnancy Risks?

There have not been clinical trials or comprehensive studies to confirm whether there are potential risks to red light therapy during pregnancy, so it's best to play it safe and don't use any phototherapy without the full support of your OB/GYN (obstetrician-gynaecologist).

There are still many unknowns, especially regarding long-term effects that relate to the eyes and the skin. "The long-term safety of these light therapies remains uncertain," says Dr. Marissa Heller, who is also a Harvard Medical School assistant dermatology professor.

In summary, there are many assurances that red light therapy, and most types of phototherapies, from blue to near-infrared, are safe. But the responsible approach is to be investigative and check things out, including whatever devices you are considering, and who will be administering the therapy, if not being self-administered at home. If there is any doubt, check with your doctor.

Phototherapy: Cause or Cure

Much of our focus on the benefits of red light therapy and other types of phototherapies has been on skin-related issues and their treatment. There are opportunities for light therapy that are controversial; does RLT cause or cure certain conditions?

Cancer: Cause or Cure

There is nothing more fearsome to people than the thought of doing something that causes cancer, and based on what has been said in the media about sunlight causing skin damage that can evolve into cancer, it is to be expected that any light treatment can raise anxiety. This applies to all types of light therapy, even though the risk of causing skin cancer is limited to UVA and UVB light; most people don't know or understand that the wavelength of UV is at the opposite end of the visible light spectrum from red.

So, there is no risk of developing skin cancer from using red light therapy; or is there? Let's take a closer look.

This issue is less about causing skin cancer, and more about accelerating the growth of existing cancer cells and tumours. "There is no evidence a person can get cancer from RLT" reports Red Light Therapy Home (2021).

- However, studies, mostly on animals at this point in the research, show that RLT could "Cause existing tumours and cancer cells to grow."

- The science that explains the beneficial qualities of RLT, confirms that it promotes cell growth. Cancer cells are simply mutated human cells, which benefit from the ATP energy generated in the mitochondria for growth. Research is underway in human trials to better understand this process and its risks.

Paradoxically, light therapy is increasingly being used to treat and potentially cure cancer, as the next section explains.

Phototherapy to Treat Cancer

The benefit of using phototherapy to treat cancer cells in the skin, or close enough to the skin to be reached by near-infrared wavelengths, is that unlike radiation, chemotherapy, and surgery, healthy cells are not damaged while the cancerous cells are destroyed. But for light therapy to be effective in this role, it depends on the right wavelength and frequency. Studies to date have identified near-infrared wavelengths to be the most effective in safely destroying cancer cells without harming healthy cells.

- A promising approach, called photoimmunotherapy (PIT), combines cancer-detecting monoclonal antibodies with light-sensitive fluorescent dye; when then exposed to deep penetrating near IR waves, the cancerous cells are destroyed, and the fluorescence enables the researcher to identify which cells were destroyed (NIH, 2010).

- More recent studies and treatments use near-infrared photoimmunotherapy. This technique uses an "antibody photoabsorber conjugate". These are antibody-like particles that are injected and travel through the bloodstream to reach tumorous cells, where they then bind to receptors on the surface of the cancer cells.

- When near-infrared light is applied to the tumour, it excites the antibody particles, which forces the cancerous cells to absorb water, swell, and then burst, causing the affected cells to die. "Photoimmunotherapy is in clinical trials in patients with inoperable tumors" (NIH, 2016).

What should you do? In summing up these research findings, if you do not have skin cancer or any other type of cancer that is close to the surface of the skin, the evidence supports that you are safe using red light and near-infrared therapy. But if you have any form of cancer, entrust your care and treatment to your dermatologist, who will assess the risks, and administer the correct type of phototherapy, if appropriate.

Photosensitivity

Some of us are hypersensitive to certain stimuli; this can include being photosensitive to light, due either to natural, or inherited causes, or possibly in reaction to medicines or supplements. If there is any possibility that you have skin sensitivities to light (for example, if you are sensitive to sunlight), *Trophy Skin* (2022) recommends that you "Do a skin sensitivity test first before using any light therapy device because different individuals respond differently to light."

If you conduct a light therapy test, or begin using RLT regularly and find that your skin is becoming excessively red, irritated or sensitive to touch, or itchy, it's best to **stop the light therapy**. Once stopped, allow your skin a few hours, or up to a couple of days, to return to normal:

- If these symptoms remain, or return after you've resumed light therapy, it's time to stop exposing your skin to LED light until you've checked in with your doctor.

- Protect your eyes by not staring at the light source, just as you would not stare at the sun. Use protective goggles at all times when receiving red light therapy, as a minimum to avoid eyestrain or cause headaches, and more importantly, to avoid long-term eye damage.

- As we've mentioned, photosensitivity can be a reaction to medications you are taking, so consider checking first with your doctor to find out if the medication can make you sensitive to red light therapy.

Cause or Stop Hair Loss?

The potential benefits of red light therapy to slow or stop excessive hair loss, or to grow lost hair, have been discussed in the previous chapter ("Benefits to the Hair and Scalp.") In summary, the effects of RLT depend on the phase that each hair shaft is in:

- Healthy, growing hair is in the anagen phase; hair that is in the catagen or resting stage may remain for some time, or enter the third, telogen phase when hair falls out.

- The ability of RLT to stimulate the mitochondria in the scalp and hair follicles (from which hair shafts emerge) determines if it can keep anagen and catagen phase hair in those stages longer.

Positive results depend on the stage of hair loss: *Healthline* (2019) says, "The procedure appears to be less effective for people in the advanced stages of hair loss as opposed to those in the early stages." Follicles that have been dormant or inactive for a long time may not respond or recover.

There is no apparent risk of RLT increasing the rate of hair loss, or causing scalp and follicle damage, except in cases of sensitivity or due to excessive or intensive application.

Headaches and Migraines

This is another category of symptoms where the debate is over **cause or cure.** Does red light therapy, or any type of phototherapy, cause headaches or migraines, or can they be an effective source of relief and elimination of pain?

Let's start with normal headaches, which can be caused by stress or tension, noise, bright light, eyestrain, and many other stimuli. If a person is sensitive to light and eyestrain, the obvious answer is that any type of phototherapy will probably cause a headache or make an existing headache worse.

But we're all different, so no broad conclusions should be drawn. If you tend to get headaches easily or often, it would be best to try red light therapy a few times before making what could be an expensive purchase.

With migraines, it is even more a question of cause or cure, especially with light being a common migraine trigger, which complicates the relationship between light and migraines. "Bright lights can exacerbate migraine attacks, and aversion to light is very common during a migraine episode," says Colleen Doherty M.D., a board-certified internist, cited in *Healthline* (2021):

- "Evidence suggests that different coloured lights affect migraines differently," Dr. Dohery says.

- But in at least some cases, the effect of light therapy may actually be beneficial, and reduce the migraine pain, or knock it out altogether.

- "Light therapy is a safe and inexpensive approach that can be combined with other lifestyle habits and medical treatments to soothe migraines as well."

Often, exposure to bright light during a migraine attack can worsen the migraine itself. Research findings demonstrate that photoreceptors on the retina of the eye detect light and "Transmit signals to the cerebral cortex of the brain, where migraine pain is perceived."

If we can understand the effects of specific coloured light wavelengths on migraines, it could be the "key to unravelling how light therapy may work in alleviating this condition." Two colours—green and blue—seem of particular importance in studying migraine prevention and treatment, for very different reasons:

Green light has positive merits: It does not activate retinal pathways as much as blue or other light rays, so it is less likely to induce a migraine. Furthermore, during a migraine attack, you are less likely to experience discomfort or light sensitivity when exposed to green light. Green light is perhaps the least likely to cause migraines, and normal headaches, as well:

- Other studies have long credited **walking in natural settings**, among trees, bushes, and grass, as conducive to stress reduction; the effusive presence of the colour green in nature probably has subtle therapeutic, relaxing qualities, in addition to whatever sounds and scents of nature add to the calming effect.

Blue light has a less positive profile: It is a large component of sunlight, and the light we stare at radiates from cell phones, computer and tablet screens, flat-screen LED televisions, LED lights, and long-life fluorescent bulbs. Blue light is everywhere, and that can be a problem for those who are sensitive to migraines.

- Blue light has more energy from a higher frequency and a shorter wavelength than green or red light. Photoreceptors exhibit the highest sensitivity to blue light. This is the reason researchers believe that exposure to blue light can intensify the pain associated with migraines.

- Dr. Doherty sums up these findings "If you are considering light therapy for migraines, green light is the least likely colour to worsen or cause migraine pain and may even soothe migraine pain."

Where does this leave red light therapy? While its benefits are extensive, it does not appear that it should be used by those who tend to be sensitive to light, and for whom the light of various wavelengths can trigger headaches and migraines.

Seasonal Affective Disorder

It may be surprising to learn that changes in the seasons can bring changes in attitude and state of mind for some people. Can seasonal changes really cause depression, and can phototherapy provide relief?

Seasonal affective disorder (SAD) is definitely real; it is a "Type of depression that's related to changes in seasons—SAD begins and ends at about the same times every year," explains the Mayo Clinic (2022).

For most people who experience this condition, the symptoms of SAD begin in the fall and continue as the winter months grow colder and darker, draining their energy and inducing a sense of moodiness.

- Most people endure and their symptoms progressively lessen as the days grow longer and warmer, often resolving during the spring and summer months.

- And less frequently, SAD can occur countercyclically, starting to cause depression in the spring or early summer, and calming back down during the fall and winter months.

The Mayo Clinic advises not to ignore or brush off yearly feelings of depression as just the "winter blues" or a "Seasonal funk that you have to tough out on your own." Instead, recognise the seriousness of the condition, and "Take steps to keep your mood and motivation steady throughout the year."

Which steps should be considered? Among the treatment options for SAD, you may want to try phototherapy, either along with or instead of psychotherapy and medications. But SAD should always be taken seriously because sometimes, it can become harmful:

- **When to see a doctor.** It's normal for you to feel down on some days when it gets dark early, colder, and gloomy. "But if you feel down for days at a time and you can't get motivated to do activities you normally enjoy, see your healthcare provider," the Mayo Clinic advises.

- **Take note** if your appetite and sleep patterns changed; if you start resorting to drinking alcohol to cheer you up, or should you develop feelings of hopelessness or consider suicide, seek medical attention immediately.

Light Therapy for SAD

Using phototherapy for SAD is not necessarily the same as when treating skin disorders, for example, when the source of red light or blue light is very close to the face or area being treated.

In contrast, for SAD treatment, you are seated a few feet from a light box that is specially designed to reduce the symptoms of SAD with the appropriate wavelengths. The treatment will involve your being exposed to a bright light, usually shortly after waking up each day. Light therapy imitates natural outdoor light, and brain studies have shown that the light causes chemical changes in the brain's section linked to mood.

Many doctors, and their patients, prefer to use non-invasive, non-drug treatments, and light therapy is one of the first recommended treatments for SAD, especially the more common fall-onset version, with the darker, shorter days. Light therapy usually starts to work within several days to a few weeks, and being a natural treatment tends to cause few side effects. The

Mayo Clinic acknowledges that "Research on light therapy is limited, but it appears to be effective for most people in relieving SAD symptoms."

We'll get deeper into the types of phototherapy devices you can purchase in a later chapter, but briefly, if you need to deal with SAD, "Before you purchase a light box to prevent or treat SAD, speak with your health care provider about the best one for you."

Take the time to become familiar with the features and options so that you buy a high-quality device that's effective and safe. Also, be sure to ask about how and when to effectively and safely use your new phototherapy light box.

Infrared and Near-Infrared Light (IR)

As wavelengths grow longer on the spectrum, next after red is near-infrared (NIR) and then full infrared, which we know for its warmth-giving property. Hotels often have infrared lights in the ceiling of bathrooms, to provide instant warmth from a safe distance.

But it's the generation of warmth that can quickly become intense heat when the IR lamp is up close to the skin, which can penetrate to a greater depth than red or near IR light.

"While red LED and NIR light wavelengths pose no danger, infrared light is thermal (heat-producing) and its wavelength penetrates your skin to a much deeper level," *Red Light Therapy Home* (2022) reports. Infrared light can quickly become hot enough to damage your eyes, burn your skin, and may even cause organ damage. For these reasons, IR light is "Not readily available in at-home therapy devices," and is used "Only to treat serious diseases and conditions."

Low risk? Maybe. Various medical and health sources have varying opinions on the risks and side effects of red light therapy, assuming it is used correctly, which is an important consideration. Any product, even your kitchen appliances, is generally safe if used correctly, but can pose a considerable danger if used carelessly. (Even a microwave can cause over-zapped foods to burst into flames!)

- *Medical News Today* (2019) defines RLT as a totally natural process. "It exposes the skin to levels of light that are not harmful—unlike UV light coming from the sun."

- On this basis, there is "Virtually no risk of side-effects from undergoing RLT." However, a person who is exposed to too much of the treatment, when administered by an inexperienced practitioner, can result in cell and tissue damage.

The takeaway from these concerns is that you should either have RLT administered by a verifiably competent professional, or if you prefer to self-administer RLT, follow the instructions that come with the advice, and, ideally, do some research to better understand the safety precautions. This way, you can greatly reduce the risk of causing burns, damage to your skin, or unprotected eyes.

A Word about Electromagnetic Fields (EMFs)

Electromagnetic Fields (EMFs) are relevant to discuss when talking about RLT due to the nature of how the therapy is delivered. Before we delve into that, let's first understand what EMFs actually are:

EMFs are physical fields produced by electrically charged objects. They can be produced both naturally and artificially:

Natural Sources of EMFs:

- **The Earth:** Our planet has its own natural magnetic field, which is why compasses work. It's also how birds and other animals can use magnetoreception for navigation. The Earth's natural magnetic field is very weak, much weaker than what we're typically exposed to from electrical devices.

- **The human body:** The human body itself generates weak electric fields. For example, nerves relay signals by transmitting electrical impulses. Most biochemical reactions, from the digestion of food, to brain activity, involve the exchange or movement of electrons.

- **The Sun:** The Earth's Sun emits electromagnetic radiation that reaches Earth. This includes visible light, heat (infrared radiation), and ultraviolet radiation, which can cause sunburn.

The primary connection between EMFs and RLT involves understanding the potential exposure to **artificial EMFs** when using these devices. Most electronic devices emit some level of

EMF. The strength of these fields can vary depending on the specific device and, of course, how it's used.

Human-Made Sources of EMFs:

- **Household electricity:** Anything plugged into an electrical outlet generates an electric field simply because it's connected to the power source. When the device is turned on and electricity is flowing, a magnetic field is also produced.

- **Electronic devices:** Devices like computers, TVs, smartphones, tablets, gaming consoles, and kitchen appliances all produce EMFs when they are in use.

- **Wireless communication:** Wireless networks (Wi-Fi), cell phones, and radio and TV signals all use radio frequency (RF) EMFs to transmit data.

- **Medical and body care devices:** From red light therapy devices to electric toothbrushes and hairdryers, many personal care appliances emit EMFs.

The World Health Organization (WHO) explains that electric fields are created by differences in voltage and magnetic fields are created when the electric current flows. The EMFs produced are typically low frequency, often referred to as Extremely Low Frequency (ELF) EMFs. While high frequency EMFs, such as X-rays and gamma rays, are known to cause damage to cells in high doses, the health effects of chronic exposure to low-frequency EMFs are still being studied.

Possible health risks associated with **long term** EMF exposure include:

- **Nervous system effects:** Some studies suggest that high levels of EMF exposure can affect the nervous system and alter brain function.

- **Cancer risk:** The International Agency for Research on Cancer (IARC) has classified ELF magnetic fields as "possibly carcinogenic to humans". This is based on statistical associations found in epidemiological studies linking EMF exposure to an increased risk for childhood leukaemia.

- **Other health problems:** There is ongoing research into other potential health problems linked to high levels of EMF exposure, including reproductive issues, developmental problems, neurodegenerative diseases, and more. However, more research is needed to draw definitive conclusions.

In the context of RLT, it's important to consider the type of device used, how often it's used, the duration of each treatment session, and the distance between the device and your body. Devices that emit lower levels of EMFs are obviously considered safer. Many manufacturers work to keep EMF levels low in their RLT devices, but it's always a good idea to check the specifications before purchasing.

It is important to note that when considering any form of therapy, RLT or otherwise, which includes exposure to EMFs, it's crucial to weigh up the potential benefits against any potential risks. With that said, however, given these potential risks, it's reasonable to want to limit unnecessary exposure to EMFs when possible.

When it comes to RLT, the amount of EMF exposure can vary depending on the device. Some devices are designed to minimise EMF emissions, while others may emit higher levels. When a red light therapy brand claims that they have "ZERO EMF emissions at the minimum usage distance of four to six inches", they are indicating that their devices have been designed and tested to ensure that the amount of EMFs emitted at that distance is effectively negligible.

Such a claim, if accurate, is an important selling point. It reflects a dedication to user safety and suggests a commitment to product quality.

How is this possible? There are several strategies that manufacturers use to reduce EMF emissions in red light therapy devices:

- **Distance:** As a fundamental principle, the intensity of EMFs drops off dramatically the further you get from the source. If a device has been designed to deliver effective treatment from a distance of 4-6 inches, then the EMF levels at that distance will be much lower than they would be right up close to the device. In simple terms, a more powerful light can be used from further away. A less powerful light has to be used close up to achieve the same benefit.

- **Shielding:** Devices can be designed with shielding materials that block or reduce EMFs. Shielding can be incorporated into the casing of the device, or the wiring. For example, twisted pair wiring can help cancel out the magnetic fields produced. This is particularly important in hand-held devices.

Remember that not all devices are created equal, and not all companies test or report their EMF emissions. If you are concerned about EMF exposure, it's worth seeking out brands that prioritise low EMF emissions and that also provide transparency around their testing procedures.

Beyond buying an EMF device that minimises EMF, here's what you can do to limit your EMF exposure during your red light therapy:

- **Distance:** Remember, the strength of the EMFs diminishes rapidly with distance from the source, so one practical way to reduce your exposure to EMFs from electrical devices is to keep a reasonable distance from them when they are in use, especially if you're using them for extended periods.

- **Duration:** Limit the duration of your exposure. The shorter the time you spend near the device, the less exposure you'll have.

Flicker

Flicker refers to the rapid and repeated change in brightness of light over time. In lighting solutions like LED bulbs or screens, flicker can occur because of the way electricity is supplied to the light source. Flicker can be problematic for several reasons:

- **Visual Comfort:** Flicker can cause eye strain, headaches, and visual disturbances, especially with prolonged exposure. This can be particularly bothersome when using RLT for extended periods.

- **Photosensitive Conditions:** For individuals with certain photosensitive conditions such as epilepsy, flicker can trigger seizures or other symptoms.

- **Reduced Therapeutic Effectiveness:** For red light therapy, a stable light source is typically preferred to ensure consistent light delivery for optimal therapeutic effect. Flickering could potentially disrupt the treatment process, though more research may be needed to definitively establish the effects of flicker on photobiomodulation.

To reduce or eliminate flicker in red light therapy devices, manufacturers can employ several strategies:

- **Higher Quality Power Supplies:** A consistent, high-quality power supply can help reduce fluctuations in electrical input that can lead to flicker.

- **Flicker-Free Driver Technology:** Some LED drivers are designed to minimise flicker by managing the way power is supplied to the LEDs.

- **Pulse Width Modulation (PWM):** PWM can be used to control the intensity of LEDs without causing visible flicker. PWM involves rapidly turning the LEDs on and off at a frequency higher than the human eye can perceive.

When selecting a red light therapy device, it's worth considering whether the manufacturer has addressed flicker, especially if you're sensitive to it or plan to use the device for extended periods. Manufacturers who prioritise a flicker-free experience often state this in their product specifications or marketing materials.

RLT devices: What and where. Along with the history, science, benefits, side effects, and applications of red light therapy, you will want to know what types of devices are available to you, and where to find them. This is what we'll cover next.

Julia E. Chatwin

Chapter 5 - Getting Practical: What, Where and How

"What I love about science is that as you learn, you don't really get answers. You just get better questions." — John Green[6]

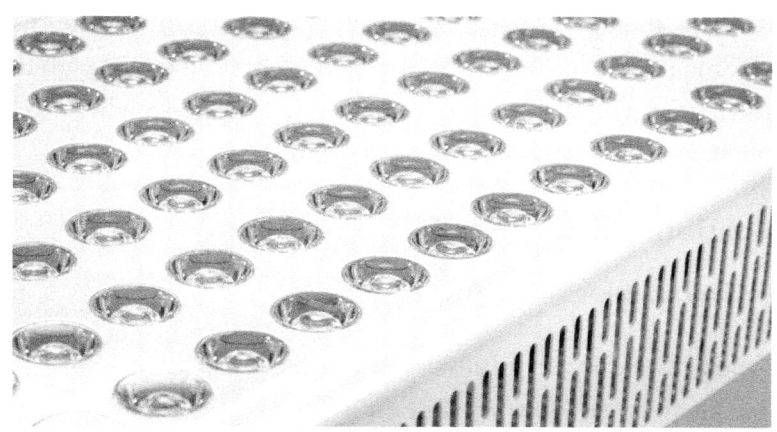

How and where you will receive your red light therapy or any other kinds of phototherapy, depends on you. Specifically:

- Your confidence in self-treating at home or wanting your applications to be performed professionally, and in a health-oriented environment.

- Your time, versus the convenience of having someone else do it all for you.

---

[6] American author

- The cost; purchasing a device for home use, for a one-time payment, or paying on a continuing, regular basis for treatments applied by others.

We'll begin by looking into the options for your RLT treatments outside the home, and then examine the many different types of red light therapy devices you can purchase for home use, including profiles of highly rated, popular brands. Armed with this information, you will be able to make the decision of where to be treated, and with what device.

Locations to Receive RLT Treatment

The Dermatologist's Office

Starting at the most professional location, you can receive red light therapy treatments at a doctor's office; various forms of light therapy have become standard practice in dermatologists' private practices. This includes not only red light therapy but also blue light therapy, administered to reduce the risk of sun damage and precancerous cells from becoming carcinomas.

In the office of a dermatologist, who is a skincare treatment doctor, you are at the lowest risk of any danger of phototherapy-induced skin damage, or eye damage. This is because of the knowledge and experience of the doctor, the professional staff, and their skill. You are also more likely to achieve the anticipated results from the therapy, since a dermatologist will manage your expectations, explaining in advance, and continuing with further treatments, what results you should—and should not—expect.

What are the **concerns** you may have about medical phototherapy treatments?

- The first to consider are the costs of a series of doctor visits, which can add up to be quite expensive over time. When you call to check if the dermatologist offers light therapy treatments, don't be afraid to ask if the treatments are covered by your health insurance (and if the office accepts your specific insurance). Even if there is insurance coverage, you may be subject to deductibles and copayments.

- You will not be able to walk in on day one and begin the light therapy; in most cases, you will be required to have an initial examination, which will lead to a diagnosis, and only then can the therapy be prescribed and scheduled. Note that having the exam is highly recommended since the dermatologist will check for precancerous cells and actual carcinomas. You should have your face, scalp, and full body checked annually.

- Finally, as with all treatments you don't do at home, there is the time and inconvenience of travel to the location, and possible waiting room time as well.

Your decision whether to receive light therapy at the dermatologist's office may be influenced by your physical condition. A serious case of acne or sun damage should sway you towards medical treatment, while less serious conditions can give you greater latitude in choosing among the options.

Other Therapy Locations

There are numerous other locations available to you for RLT; they vary greatly in their range of services and the skill and capabilities of the staff who administer the therapy.

- **Gyms, fitness centres, and saunas.** There may be a permanent setup, or an RLT specialist may be present at certain times, available by appointment, just as you can work there with a weightlifting or yoga trainer. There will usually be a private space where the therapy sessions take place.

- **Day spas, wellness centres, and skin care treatment practices.** This level of application of RLT is generally preferable to gyms and fitness centres because of the likelihood of superior quality equipment and better-trained personnel. Aestheticians (skin care practitioners) are trained and usually licensed facial care and skin care specialists who can apply phototherapy with skill.

- **Tanning salons.** Tanning salons may offer RLT in addition to customary UV exposure (which you know to avoid!). Be especially cautious and ensure there is no UV emission.

If you are considering any of these alternatives, don't assume you are risk-free; take some time to check out who will be providing the light therapy and verify their qualifications:

- Is the light-emitting equipment of high quality? Don't be afraid to ask; be sceptical and have a high standard of expectation. Remember, it's your own health and safety you need to protect.

- When choosing a clinic, make sure it's reputable and staffed by licensed professionals who are trained in red light therapy. Clinics should be clean, with well-maintained equipment, and should follow all necessary safety protocols. Don't hesitate to ask about their qualifications and experience before you book an appointment. You can obtain many benefits from red light and near-infrared light therapy from a clinic or at home, as long as it is applied safely.

RLT Devices Used Commercially

Commercial red light devices are large-scale equipment that can be used to treat a number of different conditions instead of just one.

Note: As we venture deeper into this book from here on in, I'm going to introduce specific brand names and manufacturers of RLT devices. The introduction of these is to serve purely as an aid in understanding. I would like to clearly state that, (at the time of writing at least), I hold no affiliations with any of the manufacturers or brand names mentioned in this book. My aim is, as always, to present an unbiased view of red light therapy. I encourage you to conduct further personal research when considering the purchase or use of any red light therapy device.

With that said, the Joovv 3.0 range of half or full body panels are examples of heavy-duty commercial devices with a modular design to allow the easy addition of new elements and capabilities to the device. "It is used by athletes and other people to provide pain relief as well as to treat medical conditions" (*Red Light Therapy News*).

The Rouge Curve Red Light Therapy Unit is another large-scale commercial red light therapy device that certainly would not look out of place in a dermatologists' office. The Rouge website states "Coupled with a professional motorised stand that can easily be raised, lowered and tilted into any almost position you desire, giving you the ability to customise the treatment time and distance for each patient." At $12,000, this is probably beyond the budget for most people at home.

Now it's back to you, so to speak, as we look at the light therapy equipment you can buy and use on your own.

RLT Devices to Use at Home

You can purchase devices to safely and effectively self-administer red light therapy at home, with the proper equipment, assuming it is used correctly. Be careful though, because the downside of faulty or incorrectly selected RLT devices, or their misuse, can be harmful. Fortunately, the light therapy equipment available to you for personal use, when used correctly, is a much lower-level of intensity compared to commercial devices.

Typical benefit claims for devices for use at home include "No more expensive trips to spas or expensive parlours" and "Now you can feel better within three weeks of red light therapy for the body from the comfort of home!" (Lifepro Red Light Therapy Belt, 2022).

Cost is also a key part of the decision-making process; compared to many of the professionally administered services, using a device that you own at home will be much less costly over time. For example, some spa-based treatments might add up to $1,000 or more in a year; if you cannot cover treatments in a doctor's office with health insurance, costs may add up to thousands of dollars over time.

Devices that you can purchase from retail outlets or online, and use at home, are typically priced from $50 to $500 or higher; it's a matter of size, quality of construction, types of wavelengths emitted (e.g., red only, red and near-infrared, and even more colours, like blue and white).

In the following section, there will be a brief profile of the types of red light therapy devices or products you can consider, then a presentation of the brands of devices you can purchase, and their prices. You will also find where to purchase these devices. Before we do that, we need to cover off something we've not covered yet, and that is the subject of irradiance. Let's do this now.

Remember, a well-constructed, efficient, and reliable RLT device will provide consistent and powerful therapeutic benefits over the long term. The initial cost, therefore, is not just for the device itself, but for the multitude of benefits and the potential for enhanced health and wellness it can potentially provide over time.

Irradiance

In red light therapy, irradiance is a crucial factor to consider as it directly impacts the treatment's efficacy. Irradiance, often measured in milliwatts per square centimetre (mW/cm^2), is the power density of the light being emitted by the therapy device and reaching the surface of the skin.

Here's what each part of that measurement means:

- **Milliwatt (mW):** This is a unit of power. It's one thousandth (1/1000) of a watt. The watt is the standard unit of power in the International System of Units (SI). Power represents the speed, or rate, at which energy is transferred, used, or transformed.
- **Square centimetre (cm^2):** This is a unit of area. It's used in this context to express the area over which the power (in milliwatts) is distributed.
- **Milliwatts per square centimetre (mW/cm^2):** This is a measure of power density, or how much power is distributed over a specific area.

When it comes to red light therapy, more irradiance isn't always better. The body responds best to a certain range of power densities, and exceeding this range can lead to less efficient healing or potentially even tissue damage.

Clinical studies on red light therapy have shown positive results in power densities as low as 10-100 mW/cm^2, with diminishing returns seen above levels of around 100-200 mW/cm^2. Different tissues and conditions may respond best to different irradiances, so it's always best to follow the recommendations provided by a healthcare provider or the device manufacturer.

Additionally, as discussed, the irradiance level you'll receive decreases with distance. As you move farther away from the light source, the power density decreases because it's distributed over a larger area. This is why treatment times may vary depending on how close you are to the device.

It is also important to consider the wattage of the RLT device. For example, when comparing two identical looking panels. If one panel states 300w and another just 45w, then clearly the higher wattage device has more power and is likely to deliver more light over a wider area. A higher wattage device is typically more potent and beneficial, but it's essential to understand why:

- **Power Density:** Devices with higher wattage usually have a higher power density, which means they have a larger coverage area, allowing you to treat larger parts of your body at once. This can be especially beneficial if you are looking to conduct full-body treatments.
- **Treatment Time:** Because high-wattage devices emit more light, they often require less treatment time compared to lower-wattage devices. As you can achieve the desired dose of red light therapy in a shorter amount of time, it can make the therapy more convenient.
- **Depth of Penetration:** Higher power/irradiance can also lead to a deeper penetration of light, potentially leading to more profound therapeutic effects. The light from higher wattage devices can reach deeper tissues, which can be beneficial if you're aiming to target not just skin but also muscles, joints, or other deep tissues.

While the wattage of a red light therapy device is an important factor to consider, especially for larger panels, it is not as crucial for smaller handheld devices intended for targeted treatment.

Here's why:

- **Targeted Treatment:** Handheld devices are usually designed for localised treatment rather than full-body exposure. They focus on specific areas, like the face or a particular joint or muscle group, so they do not necessarily need the high wattage required by larger panels to cover a broader area.
- **Close Proximity Use:** These devices are often used in close proximity to the skin, which can maximise the light absorption even with a lower wattage.
- **Extended Use Time:** Since handheld devices are often applied to a smaller area, extended use time is typically more manageable. While high-wattage devices deliver therapeutic light dosage more quickly, using a lower wattage device for a longer duration can still provide effective treatment.
- **Safety and Comfort:** Lower wattage devices also generate less heat and are generally safer and more comfortable for close-up, targeted treatments.

That said, even for handheld devices, it's crucial to ensure that the device offers the correct therapeutic wavelengths, and it adheres to safety standards. As always, follow the manufacturer's instructions for use to get the best results safely.

In summary, understanding irradiance and wattage (the power of the device) is key in red light therapy as it determines the dosage of light you receive during a treatment session. This, in turn, has a direct influence on the therapy's effectiveness.

Examples of RLT Devices for Home Use

The following brands are examples of what is currently available for home use and are profiled to include the positioning, or overall brand promise, a brief summary of its technology and wavelengths provided, and primary benefits. As you will see, some devices provide both red light and near-infrared light options; others provide only red light. Some provide additional spectrums of light.

You will see here presented different types of devices, from tabletops to wearable belts. This will give you a good idea of what's "out there".

During the research phase of this book, certain red light therapy devices emerged as particularly noteworthy due to the high praise they received in numerous online reviews. They are presented here to illustrate the range of options available in the current market (2023). Again, I am not recommending or endorsing any particular brand or product here. In making your evaluation and eventual decision, consider the product type, the light wavelengths each provides, the power, and whether multiple wavelengths (if available) can be emitted only individually or combined to provide more benefits in a shorter time. This list of products is by no means exhaustive.

Product Example 1

Bestqool Half-Body Red Light Therapy Pro100

This first product is typical of a panel format; the device stands on a table, shelf, or counter, and is covered with LED lights.

- This device is positioned as "especially effective for boosting skin health and increasing collagen" and has the "ability to penetrate deeper into the tissue, joints and organs, making it ideal for enhancing muscle recovery, reducing joint pain and inflammation." There are three levels of therapy: red light, which helps boost skin health and increase collagen production; near-infrared light provides deep penetration to tissues and aids muscle restoration; and combined red and near-red therapy for optimum benefit and effect.

- The device is equipped with 100 dual-chip LEDs, emitting both red light and near-infrared light. The product states that for optimal results, it is to be used for 10-25 minutes per session. It's a compact, rectangular table top unit, measuring 19.6 x 8.3 x 3.1 inches, and weighing 9.2 lbs. The unit weighs 9.2 pounds, consumes approximately 165 watts and is designed for longevity, stating a lifespan of over 30,000 hours. The device is backed by a 2-year warranty for peace of mind.

- The product page states that this unit provides an irradiance of 94mw/cm^2 when used at a distance of 6 inches making this unit very powerful indeed.

- It also states that there are no detectable EMF emissions at a distance of 5 inches.

The brand is available at Amazon, retailing for around the $329.99 price point. You can also buy directly from their website.

Bestqool offers a range of lights to suit all purposes.

Product Example 2
The BIO 300 Red Light Therapy device by Platinum Lights

- Delivering an impressive 300w of power across its 100 x 3w LEDs, this device is compact and robust looking, with dimensions measuring 19" x 9" x 3". Similar to the Bestqool it would fit well into a living or office space. This unit also states an irradiance of 94mw/cm^2 when used at a distance of 6 inches.

- First off, its coverage area is large (like the Bestqool), making it suitable for treating large sections of the body. One of the most striking features is the BIO 300's robust temperature handling. At a maximum of 130°F (55°C), it holds steady under extensive usage without compromising the integrity of the unit. This is thanks to the dual built-in cooling fans—showing a commitment to product durability and user safety.

- The advertised lifespan of the BIO 300's LED bulbs is impressive at 100,000 hours. If accurate, this longevity translates to significant value for the price and is a sure sign of quality.

- Electromagnetic field (EMF) emission is another important aspect to consider, especially for health-conscious users. The BIO 300 promises "Zero EMF at 6", which should provide users with peace of mind regarding any potential EMF exposure risks.

- The BIO 300 also comes with a generous 3-year warranty, underscoring the manufacturer's confidence in the product's quality and durability.

This panel currently retails for $399.00, available directly from Platinum Lights.

This is just one of many products from Platinum Lights.

Product Example 3

Infraredi Flex Lite

- Weighing in at a light 3.5 kgs, the Infraredi Flex Lite Red Light Therapy Device combines portability with power, featuring 60 x 3-watt LEDs and offering an output of 180 watts.

- The device boasts a no-flicker design, which minimises potential eye strain or discomfort during use and reports zero EMF at a 5cm distance.

The product is available directly from their website and retails for $379.

Again, this is just one of many products from Infraredi.

Wearable Red Light Therapy Devices

Red Light Therapy News (2022) cites the progress within the phototherapy industry; it has grown at a brisk pace, with the devices becoming smaller, portable and hand-held, and more localised. "Most Red Light Therapy devices can now be worn", as this belt demonstrates:

Lifepro Red Light Therapy Belt, described as "Near-Infrared Light Therapy & Red Light Therapy for Relaxing Muscle, Inflammation, and Improved Circulation."

- Users can choose between two LED settings: red light therapy, which is known for the ability to improve the health and appearance of skin tissue; near-infrared light penetrates to reach deeper tissues and helps in relaxing muscles.

- The red light therapy belt is long enough to wrap around the body and states that it fits comfortably while the user sits, lies down, or walks around, leaving their hands free. The user simply has to remove jewellery before beginning the light therapy.

- Weighing just 1.1 lbs, the therapy belt is small enough and light so it can be rolled up to fit in a small carrying bag when not in use; it would tuck away easily in a drawer. The Lifepro therapy belt comes with a remote control that plugs into your computer's USB port, or an electrical outlet to recharge.

This product is available at around $160 from the manufacturer's website.

Omnilux Contour Face

Here's another different form of RLT. The following device covers the full spectrum of visible light therapy and is a facial mask:

- Designed specifically for facial treatment, weighing in at a mere 330g for both the mask and controller.
- Emits both red and near-infrared light at wavelengths of 633nm and 830nm, respectively.
- Flexible silicone design.
- The recommended usage schedule is clearly defined, suggesting three to five 10-minute treatments per week for an initial period of four to six weeks.
- A gentle wipe-down after use keeps it clean and ready for the next session.

The Omnilux Contour Face is undoubtedly a high-quality device offering targeted red and near-infrared light therapy for facial skin rejuvenation.

Price at $395 and available directly from their website.

Other examples

In addition to the masks and belts among the above products, other examples include:

- The "reVive Light Therapy DPL II Full-Face LED Light Therapy," which is worn on the face, to treat facial issues, from acne and spots to dry, inflexible skin and wrinkles.

- "Nushape Lipo Wrap," which is a belt that is worn on the arm, leg, or waist for localised fat reduction, along with any skin problems to treat.

- The "iRestore Laser Hair Growth System" is designed like a helmet. As the name states, its light waves target dormant (catagen phase) hair follicles to stimulate anagen phase hair growth.

- OMNILUX Contour Glove, a treatment specifically for hands; an "FDA-cleared, dermatologist-recommended red light therapy device with clinically-proven results for skin rejuvenation." The hand is inserted into the glove, where the lights are placed. It's at the higher end of the costs at $345.

Handheld LED Devices

Handhelds offer specific localised applications, and given their small size and relatively low power levels, they tend (in most cases) to be a low-cost way to break into the use of red light and near-infrared light therapy devices. Also, people who may prefer not to expose larger areas to light waves can achieve a targeted application by treating a limited region.

For example, the benefits of localised treatment for users of handhelds include:

- Skincare treatment, including facial care. Specific problem areas can be locally treated, like a single blemish or spot, or individual acne pimples, without having to expose their full face.

- Athletic performance and post-workout recovery, especially for pain reduction through targeted treatment of joints and muscles. The lactate that accumulates in muscle tissue and causes stiffness and soreness may be dissipated.

- Wound healing can be localised to the injured area to increase blood circulation that more effectively brings oxygen and nutrients and carries away metabolic waste. Hypertrophy, the repair of muscle tissues by hard exercise, can be accelerated.

Examples of handheld light therapy devices, listed as highly rated by *Forbes* (2021):

The Pure Daily Care Luma Light Therapy Wand

Described as a sophisticated handheld device with 4-in-1 capabilities. The Luma wand works as light therapy for skincare, but it also massages, firms wrinkles, and provides lifting action. This device emits three different wavelengths: red, blue, and green light (more on this later), which can be applied individually or in combination for optimal effects in less time. It's at the higher end in cost at $345.

Project E Beauty Light Therapy Device

Described as "Intense, powerful LED light therapy," This handheld wand device consists of 40 red LED diodes that "pack a powerful dose of red light, which can boost collagen, elastin, and other compounds that lead to a better complexion."

A unique feature is the option to choose between a continuous flow of light or a pulse mode that emits brief but powerful bursts of therapeutic light. It operates at a wavelength of 630 nm. Stated benefits include skin tightening and removing wrinkles, collagen increase, and increased elasticity.

Exerscribe RedTonic Light Therapy Wand

This compact handheld resembles a small, cylindrical flashlight, but it's loaded with "Intense LED diodes; you'll be amazed at how bright and effective the device is." It comes complete with protective glasses and a cleaning kit, and is powered by rechargeable batteries for complete portability. It provides three wavelengths of therapeutic red light: 630 nm, 660 nm, and 850 nm, and is beneficial for relieving pain and for targeted, localised skin care.

LightStim LED Therapy Device: This handheld wand is especially recommended for treating acne and is described as a "Powerful, effective, and natural solution to clearer skin." It works to calm down existing acne breakouts and destroy most of the acne-causing bacteria to prevent acne pimples from breaking out on the skin. The wand's effectiveness is based on both red light and blue light wavelengths, which "Work together synergistically for a more radiant, youthful appearance." For best results with stubborn cases of acne, daily application is recommended. It's available for the price of $249.

ReVive Light Therapy Wand: A "Lux Collection Clinical LED Light Therapy Tool." This lightweight, handheld device provides infrared, red, blue, and amber wavelengths for versatile, deep-penetrating light (DPL) skin therapy. This product is available for $149.

- It is "Intended for treatment of wrinkles, acne, and inflammation associated with acne." It uses light-emitting diodes (LEDs) to release the wavelengths that most effectively help improve and heal your skin.

- "Setting one features red, infrared, and amber lights for anti-aging," by reducing fine lines and wrinkles, helps to reverse sun damage, and "Promotes healing for younger-looking skin with improved texture and tone."

- "Setting two features blue and red lights for acne treatment," by targeting and wiping out bacteria that cause breakouts.

- "Setting three features the synergistic combination of red, infrared, amber, and blue light" wavelengths for both anti-ageing and acne treatment, saving time and optimising results.

Where to Buy

These, and many other handheld red light therapy devices are usually available at department stores, like Nordstroms, Macy's, and other big retailers like Walmart, Walgreens, Target, Bed, Bath & Beyond, CVS, Rite-Aid, and their websites where you can order online.

In addition, as mentioned earlier, the online market for handhelds, and all other types and forms of light therapy brands are available from online companies, notably Amazon and other large online retailers.

Red Light Therapy Beds

Phototherapy beds are no longer limited to tanning beds! LED red light therapy beds are a newly emerging part of the market, albeit not yet deeply penetrating the at-home segment. Red light therapy beds started to become available to the public when the "LightStim LED bed" was given clearance by the FDA in 2017.

Unlike the medically discouraged tanning beds, the red light therapy beds are considered safe and without the risks of tanning beds, given the differences in technologies and the wavelengths involved: red light beds are free of the risky UVA and UVB waves used by tanning beds.

- "Red light therapy beds have been shown to lower your blood pressure, help the body heal, rejuvenate the skin, ward off acne and fine lines and help with hair growth," *Red Light Therapy News* reports.

The at-home market for light therapy beds is limited for now, due to the size and cost of the units—they take up quite a bit of room, compared to the small screens, masks, and belts in use today. For now, their use is largely confined to commercial locations; gyms, spas, salons, wellness centres, and skin care treatment practices where commercial light therapy treatments are already being performed.

The 5 Biggest Buying Mistakes

Here are the 5 biggest mistakes that people make when buying an RLT device. If you heed this advice, you will be on the right track.

Mistake 1: Ignoring the Wavelength Specifications

One of the most crucial factors when purchasing a red light therapy device is the wavelength of light it emits. Not all devices offer the optimal wavelengths (around 660nm for red light and 850nm for near-infrared light) that have been shown in studies to have therapeutic benefits. Purchasing a device that does not emit light within these ranges might lead to ineffective treatment.

Mistake 2: Choosing Price Over Quality

As we have seen, RLT devices can vary greatly in price. While it may be tempting to go for the cheapest option, lower-priced devices often have lower power output, less coverage area, and may not deliver the desired results. Always look for a balance between cost and quality, and remember, investing in a good device can save money in the long run. Remember the "buy cheap, buy twice" adage. It's best to get it right the first time!

Mistake 3: Not Considering Treatment Area Size

Red light therapy devices come in different sizes, from handheld devices to large panels. If you're planning to treat a small area, such as your face, a smaller device may be suitable. However, if you want to treat larger areas, or your whole body, you will need a larger device or panel. Choosing the wrong size for your needs could result in inefficient treatment.

Mistake 4: Neglecting to Check Warranty and Return Policy

As with any significant purchase, it's essential to look at the warranty and return policy. A device might look good on paper, but every individual's response to red light therapy can vary. It is prudent to choose a device that comes with a solid warranty and a fair return policy, in case the device doesn't work as expected or has any issues.

Mistake 5: Overlooking FDA Clearance

In the United States, it's crucial to check whether the red light therapy device is FDA cleared. An FDA-cleared device has been evaluated for safety and effectiveness. Using a device that hasn't been approved could potentially be risky.

A Perspective from the Cleveland Clinic (2022)

Are Devices Purchased for At-Home Use a Safe, Reasonable Option?

You can find a large selection of red light and near-infrared therapy products if you search online. "While these products are generally safe to use, they may use a lower wavelength frequency (meaning they're less powerful) than devices that may be used by dermatologists or other trained skin professionals". Therefore, in some cases, you may not get the results you are expecting.

"If you do choose to purchase a red light therapy device, make sure to shield your eyes for protection, follow all directions and take good care of the device."

In addition to applications available through dermatologists and other medical offices (at one extreme), and home use (at the other extreme), you may find phototherapy being offered and promoted at saunas and beauty salons, tanning salons, gyms and fitness centres, facial care spas, and wellness centres.

- "Be cautious of who is supplying and where you are receiving treatment. It's always best to check in with a medical professional about the best options to treat your skin condition."

The timeless phrase, "Better safe than sorry" comes to mind. Especially when it comes to ordering products on the internet, when persuasive advertising, sale prices, and free shipping can easily compel us to make a few quick clicks, and the product is on its way.

Resist being compulsive and hesitate long enough to at least do some research to learn more, especially from unbiased sources like blogs and rating sites, where you may see actual customer comments, both positive and negative. Then, armed with the facts, and shielded from overly enthusiastic ad copy, you can more confidently proceed with your decision and action.

Use at Home. In the next two chapters, we are going to follow up the review of products you can purchase to use at home, and the caution from the Cleveland Clinic, with practical advice on how to use RLT safely and to full effectiveness. We'll include not just red light and near-infrared light, but white, blue, green, yellow and cyan light. All of which have specific applications and potential benefits.

Julia E. Chatwin

Chapter 6 - Using Red Light Therapy at Home

"The beauty and the scent of roses can be used as a medicine and the sun rays as a food." — Nikola Tesla[7]

Frequently Asked Questions to Cover the Basics

You expect great results from the red light therapy device you have purchased (or are planning to buy soon; maybe today); you may be hoping to clear up stubborn acne, get rid of dark spots, scars, or blemishes, diminish the appearance of fine lines and wrinkles, reduce pain, treat stiff or sore joints and muscles, stop hair loss, or lower the frequency and intensity of migraines.

Or perhaps you are hoping to gain several of those benefits, or maybe even all of them.

When it comes to red light and near-infrared devices for your personal use at home, you've come to the point in the decision-making process where you naturally have questions and concerns that need to be addressed and answered. This chapter is organised into a series of frequently asked questions, which cover the basics of everything you need to know.

Frequently Asked Questions About Safety

Q: Is red and near-infrared light therapy safe?

---

[7] Serbian-American inventor

You may have heard enough, and read enough, to be a bit anxious about safety; or maybe you are more than a little concerned. This is the right approach; to address your concerns rather than worrying if you've made a mistake and have taken on a responsibility you can't handle. You may have these issues in mind:

Q: Will you burn your face? Or can you damage your eyes and hurt your vision? Or can your light therapy treatment cause skin cancer?

Q: You've learned that red and near-infrared are at light wavelengths that actually penetrate the epidermis outer skin and below, through the subcutaneous dermis layer. But can subcutaneous deep penetration also be a bad thing?

Q: Should you limit your light therapy treatment to professionals? Or skip the matter altogether and seek other types of treatment?

Q: Are there side effects from using red light and near-infrared light therapy, even if you are careful??

The answers to these questions are at once positive, but conditional:

- For safe and effective red light and near-infrared light therapy, you need to use good quality equipment, in a form that is designed to treat the area where you need it. It makes good sense, for example, to acquire a mask or screen to treat facial problems or a glove for your hands; while a belt would be completely inappropriate. Conversely, muscular and joint problems are well treated by belts and handhelds that can reach and concentrate wavelengths where needed.

- And equally important, it's up to you to operate your light therapy correctly, and that requires carefully following the instructions that are included with the device. Do not treat your new device casually, by assuming you just need to plug it in, turn it on, and start your treatments. It's not another iPhone, video screen, or set of Bluetooth AirPods in-ear speakers; it's a powerful high-energy emitting machine, even if it's a small handheld or tabletop model that has a lower intensity to the one that the dermatologist uses.

- There are no known side effects from red and near-infrared wavelength therapy if the devices are being used correctly, according to the directions provided with the device. But there can be reactions if certain medications are being taken; that is why it's a smart move to check with your doctor before beginning RLT therapy.

- Red light therapy is classified as non-invasive and isn't harsh to the skin. However, if eye protection is not worn when using the device, there are real risks that there can be damage to the eyes. There are also potential risks of skin damage if you place yourself too close to the device.

- To borrow the recommendation from the Cleveland Clinic at the end of the previous chapter.

- "If you do choose to purchase a red light therapy device, make sure to shield your eyes for protection, follow all directions and take good care of the device."

- Long-term safety and potentially harmful effects of using red and near-infrared light therapy have not yet been determined.

To sum it up, most light therapy devices are safe and beneficial for you to use at home if operated responsibly. But what does "operated responsibly" really mean? That's what we'll be covering in a section about questions you may have about how to safely and effectively use your new light therapy device, but first, let's discuss how you can select the right one for what you need.

Frequently Asked Questions About Selection

It may be tempting to select a phototherapy device because it looks great online (or in a store), or because it promises to treat and cure everything. But remind yourself there are many aspects of the decision you need to weigh, and the first among them is what you plan to use it for.

Q: How to begin? What kind of phototherapy devices should be considered for you to use unsupervised, at home?

Q: What types of devices should you consider, from the extensive range of red light therapy devices that are available?

Q: There are multiple wavelength options being offered; should you choose red or other options, like near-infrared?

The answers to these questions can be summed up: "Choose a device size and type that targets your treatment goals," *WikiHow* (2022) advises. Be objective in deciding what you need your RLT device to do, and recognise that no single device should be expected to do everything:

- You can depend on using small standing devices or portable handhelds for facial care and face skin rejuvenation; to slow hair loss and stimulate new hair growth; and to promote healing and reduce pain in the muscles, knees, wrists, elbows, hips, and feet. You can probably reach your shoulders for treatment if your joints are not too tight, and you have a good range of movement.

- "Many devices are made for specific areas of your body, such as red light therapy masks that target your face." For the hands, there are RLT gloves, with LED lights inside. In selecting these highly specialised types of devices, you may experience optimal benefits, but cannot use the device for treating other parts of the body.

- Larger, full-body devices cover a lot of skin surface at once, although the intensity at any given place may be less than a handheld or specialised device can focus on. Large devices work best for "Chronic inflammation and body pain, muscle recovery, weight loss, and improving blood flow and circulation" (*WikiHow*).

- Multi waves? As you will have seen in the previous chapter, some devices may offer only red light therapy;

others may provide both red and near-infrared wavelengths. With some devices that provide both wavelengths, you may only use each one independently; but other devices may allow the two wavelengths to be combined to work together, achieving greater intensity and synergy.

- Consider if you would prefer that the device you select provides both red light and near-infrared light options to optimise the benefits of your red light therapy.

Frequently Asked Questions About How to Operate Your Device

You've taken your light therapy device out of the box, and now what? You want to start using it as soon as you can; after all, the faster you get going, the faster you'll see results, right? Well, in principle, that's true, but let's pause for a reality check: As you will learn in the next section about other concerns, you will need to have patience, because red and near-red infrared light therapy take time to work; they are not an instant fix:

Your priority at this moment should be spending some time learning how to use your device. This will go a long way in helping you to "do it right," and ensure safe, effective operations. This leads us to the first question:

Q: You now have your device, and you've opened the box; what should you do first?

- Take a moment to make sure everything that should be in the box is there; nothing is missing or appears broken.

- Now take out the instructions and read them fully and completely. This is how you will learn to set up the specific device; how to charge it up (if it's rechargeable); where to place it (if it's not portable or specific to your face or hand); how to store it; and of the greatest importance; how to use it correctly.

- Pay close attention to the distance you need to have the device from your skin; how long to expose the light in each treatment session; how many sessions you should have in a week; and for how many weeks. Each brand and type of device will have its own unique instructions; but as a starting point, the following question provides general or typical instructions.

Q: How long should your red light therapy sessions be for maximum effectiveness? What is the optimal exposure time for both effectiveness and safety?

- "How long" depends on where you are in terms of the length of time you have been applying the treatments. Begin with 10-minute treatments, and skip a day; that is, apply the therapy every other day. Then start to work your way up after three or four sessions, to applications lasting 15 to 20 minutes, but maintain the frequency of applying every other day.

- Be consistent. Stick with 3 to 4 sessions a week, following the every-second-day protocol. Don't extend the length of the next session if you have missed a session; you can't make it up safely and might risk burning or skin damage. Maintaining your therapy sessions for the same amount of time, and for the same number of days per week, is the way you will get the best results, and not by longer or more frequent light therapy sessions.

- Find a time, preferably during the morning or evening, when you can complete your sessions without disturbance or interruption.

Beyond these general guidelines, follow the instructions supplied with the device, which will be more specific about the timing and frequency of the sessions. In time, you may be able to apply the light therapy every day, or two sessions per day at 10 minutes each time, but be alert to discomfort or reddening:

When you are first starting red and near-infrared light therapy, the areas being treated may feel warm. That's normal and not a concern, but if you have sensitive skin, or the treated areas are a deep red and the skin feels tight, ease back on the length of your session, and make sure you are not too close to the device.

If you are uncertain about your sensitivities, it is advisable to conduct a patch test on a small area of your skin before proceeding to larger areas, just to see how your skin responds.

For ease of application, select an appropriate location to use your device; a place where you can stand or sit for up to 20 minutes at a time, and not be disturbed. It's a good idea to spruce up the area to make it relaxing; you can do this with music, aromatherapy, and candles. Some people find this time to be good for meditation.

Distance

Ensure you position yourself at a sufficient distance from the device, typically 6 inches or more, to be outside of the magnetic field. However, aim to be as close as feasible to minimise losses due to beam angle and skin reflection.

If you notice considerable heat or warmth on your skin during use, adjust your distance, moving further away until the warmth becomes subtle.

For skin treatments and sensitive areas, maintaining a greater distance is recommended. Conversely, for deeper treatment, position yourself closer to the device. In time, you will naturally know what works best for you.

Frequently Asked Questions About Other Concerns

You are being cautious, careful, and curious. You want to know all you can about using electromagnetic radiation in light wavelengths to achieve your health, fitness, and appearance goals. So far, we've covered much of what you need to know. Here are a few more questions you may have.

Q: Is the device approved by a responsible authority?

- You will considerably reduce the risks of manufacturing defects or unsafe operations if the device has been cleared by the FDA. This means the manufacturer has submitted the device for laboratory testing by an independent service.

- Be alert to cheaply priced devices costing well below the normal range; for example, available for $12.99 or $15.99 from a company you've never heard of, or who has no website (or a tacky, cheap-looking site).

- Heads up too that any eBay seller is a real vendor with thousands of likes, and not an individual trying to sell one or two devices they have. Verify that the company offers a satisfaction guarantee.

Q: How much should the RLT device cost; do you have to spend a lot for a safe, quality unit?

- Red light therapy devices can be priced from about $50 to over $1,000, with many reputable models available in the $100 to $399 range. The pricing is affected by many factors: Depending on their size; quality of construction; scope of wavelengths provided (red only, or red plus near-infrared); and the types of controls and timers. Accessories provided can also affect pricing.

- As you can see from the pricing, the cost of owning and using home devices is far less than receiving regular professional treatments, which can add up to $1,000 or $2,000 annually.

Q: Are at-home red light therapy devices as effective as professional ones?

- In a word, no. This is not surprising and should be viewed positively, for safety concerns, at least. "At-home devices are less powerful than professional ones," WikiHow assures us since we're not professionals with the training and access to powerful equipment.

- In today's fast-paced world, our desire for instant gratification has been perpetuated by our ability to have purchases delivered at the tap of a screen or get answers to questions within seconds. Sometimes, the most rewarding experiences in life come from practices that require time, patience, and perseverance. Endeavours that call for us to slow down, persist, and appreciate the journey are often the most rewarding. We need to practise the lost art of patience! You can still have the same beneficial results if you simply have the patience to wait a little longer! "In general, you have to complete more sessions with an at-home device to see the same results that you would with an in-office device." Why? Professional devices are more effective because they can emit higher light frequencies than the FDA would clear for home use. So, it just takes longer, but you'll get there.

- But if you are impatient and want faster results, attend several professional therapy sessions, and then switch over to your at-home phototherapy device to continue to improve your results.

Q: How long do you need to wait to see results?

- It depends. In most cases, it may take up to 8 to 12 weeks, especially for "hard cases," like stubborn acne, fine lines and wrinkles, sun damage and dark spots, and muscular and joint injuries. But many conditions, like soreness and aches, and even migraines, may respond far sooner.

- As WikiHow explains, "Red light therapy works at the cellular level, meaning that the process of healing, improving collagen production, and reducing inflammation take time."

However, there are many reports of near-term or even immediate improvements, especially to the skin and deeper, subcutaneous tissues. But the best plan is to manage your expectations and give your red light therapy the time it needs.

Q: How can you keep track of your phototherapy progress?

- One easy way to record your progress with skin treatments is to take photos once a week of the treatment area. You may not be able to observe the before-and-aftereffects just by looking, but over time, the photos will provide a realistic "progress report."

- But be sure to take the photos in the same location, especially with the same lighting conditions, so there are no biases introduced into the evaluation. You may not see big differences at first, or from week to week, but after several weeks or a month or two, comparing the starting (pre-treatment) photo with the latest should show satisfying progress.

- If you are using red and near-infrared light therapy for non-visible benefits, like helping muscles and joints to recover, or to reduce pain, maintain a journal to record how you feel each week. For pain, you can rate the pain on a scale of 1 to 10; for tight or stiff muscles and joints, you may use a 10-point scale to assess the range of movement.

How to Avoid Mistakes Using Red Light and Near-Infrared Therapy at Home

Using your device correctly and as instructed is the way to get the best results while ensuring your safety. While effectiveness and safety have been emphasised throughout this chapter, and throughout the entire book, this is a series of reminders that can serve as a checklist of good practices. Read them now and refer back periodically to refresh yourself. It is easy to make mistakes, especially if you are rushed, or impatient, and want results sooner than realistic.

Manage your expectations and behaviour, and all will work out. Your device, whether you've purchased it for face care or sore muscles; back pain, or stretch marks and scars, will only be as good as how well it is operated.

Select carefully. Obtain and use the correct device for what you require. The advertising for the various light therapy devices can be tempting, and you can be tempted to buy one that looks great, without carefully considering your specific needs.

- Do you have room in your home for a large device, or can you make good use of a smaller device? A device that can target your face or other specific areas that would benefit from treatment.

- Conversely, to cover large areas of your body, such as for fibromyalgia or sciatica, or your full legs, a large screen-type device may be better for full coverage, for a shorter time. You need to balance needs with the practicality of usage and storage.

Respect distance. Use your device at the correct distance for the best effects, without risking burns or soreness. According to *Red Light Therapy News* (2022) editor Emma Williams, this requires some experimentation on your part, because the science of ideal distances between the skin and body is not yet complete.

- Her recommendation is that from 6 to 12 inches is the range where deep penetration is desired (especially if near-infrared is applied), and from 12 up to 36 inches for surface skin treatments.

- Admittedly, these are wide ranges of distance, so take the conservative route and start out on the more distant options, and gradually try moving closer, as long as there's no burning or excess reddening of the skin.

Stay hydrated, at all times, especially when conducting red light and near-infrared therapy. Drinking the proverbial eight glasses of water a day may not be mandatory, but it's known that your cells need water continually for metabolism and other processes.

- New studies have found that keeping the cells fully hydrated can increase the energy production that red light and near-infrared therapy can stimulate.

Be consistent with your treatments for the best effects. Unlike having scheduled treatment sessions at a doctor's office or spa, with at-home treatments you are on your own to conduct—or miss—your sessions. These should, ideally, be performed on a regular basis, like every other morning or evening. As we've mentioned, it is not responsible to make up missed sessions with extra sessions, or longer than normal sessions.

- Set up a schedule that you can follow; it should be at the same time (for example 7:00 AM), and when you will not be interrupted or be obliged to be somewhere else. Early mornings and late evenings tend to be safe times to schedule.

Use the appropriate wavelength settings. You may think that near-infrared (NIR) and red light perform the same or similar functions, but there are important differences, which affect how each is to be used:

- Red light is more effective than NIR in treating topical skin issues, growth, or regrowth of hair, and in healing small wounds.

- NIR can probe deeply into and beneath the skin, so it can be used to treat subcutaneous pain relief in muscles and joints, deep healing, and (potentially) cognitive health.

Understand the settings. Different devices will have their own particular settings, for red light and for NIR light, and if appropriate, a dual setting to provide a combination of both wavelengths. In many cases, you may switch between these three settings by using the mode button to make your selection.

- It's okay to use the dual setting, especially if you're not sure about which is best for your condition, or to treat unknown issues with the synergistic effect of the two wavelengths. (FYI, near-infrared light is just outside the visible spectrum, so you should not expect to see it working visibly like red light.)

Do not block or interfere with the direct contact of light therapy on your skin. You may use sunblock to prevent UV sun damage, but it will also block many other wavelengths, including red and near-infrared; this will render the treatment ineffective.

- This is another incentive to conduct your treatments early in the morning before sunblock or any skincare creams or lotions are applied. Be sure as well not to block the rays with clothing; NIR might penetrate some fabrics, but red can't.

Involve your doctor. Be sure to discuss your use (or plan to use) red light and near-infrared light therapy with your medical practitioner. Although applying these light therapies at home is recognised for being non-invasive, drug-free, safe, and painless qualities, speaking with your doctor is strongly recommended.

- Among the reasons to check in is to ensure you are not taking any medications that might be affected by the wavelength activity. Or, during pregnancy, there could be effects that are not yet known, and unnecessary risks are to be avoided. By keeping your doctor in the loop, you can be assured that you can make the right decisions for your health and safety.

Respect your schedule. As noted above, it's recommended that you make a schedule for your treatments and stick to it. There are good reasons: You'll make faster progress, without risks of skin damage, as compared to haphazard scheduling, with missed sessions, or sessions that are cut short due to other urgencies. You are discouraged from trying to make up for missed therapy sessions.

- "Even though this practice is not particularly dangerous and harmful to the user, it should be noted that red light therapy doesn't operate in that manner," *Red Light Therapy News* (2022) advises, and adds that "Skipping sessions and trying to pack all the missed ones into one session will actually make the therapy less effective, so this should be avoided."

Give it time. Some red light therapy users make the mistake of raising their expectations for the results; they expect too much, too soon. Red light and near-infrared light therapy have earned a reputation as positive, safe methods for providing effective cures and treatments for a range of health problems. "However," Emma Williams notes, "It is not and can never be a miracle cure."

- It is not a one-time or occasional treatment, but instead is "Highly recommended that it be frequently and consistently used. This is because it is very possible for the issue it was used to treat to return after stoppage." This therapy is a continuous activity, which takes perseverance, patience, and the discipline of sticking to a schedule and respecting the timing and distance of application. Stay calm and stay with it!

Note your progress. There's nothing as motivating and encouraging as seeing and feeling the results of your treatment with red light and near-infrared therapy. This includes relieving the pain and discomfort of arthritis and sore joints and muscles, and reduction of acne, blemishes, dark spots, and other skin disorders. But there's a catch: You'll need to do some tracking to accurately measure the positive changes you are experiencing.

- As noted in the previous section, you can take photos of the treated skin area, starting before treatment begins, and continuing on a regular basis, like every week, or every other week. Don't expect daily or early results, but after a few weeks or a month, there should be evidence of reduced reddening, shrinking of acne zits, and lightening of dark spots. For more internal issues, you can keep a log of pain and discomfort levels.

Protect your eyes. Yes, we've been saying this repeatedly, but with good reason. You don't have to be reminded of how precious your vision is, and no treatment is worth the risk of causing eye damage. Fortunately, red and near-infrared light do not pose the serious risks of UVA and UVB rays, which are at the opposite end of the visible and near visible light spectrum; UV rays are harmful because of their shorter, more penetrating wavelength, and the intensity of their much higher frequency.

- But too much of anything can pose risks if used carelessly, and to excess. So simply follow the guidelines first, never look directly into the light-emitting lamps, and second, use goggles whenever you are undergoing light therapy treatment. Usually, a protective goggle is included with the red light therapy device, and "It is highly recommended that these goggles be used anytime you want to use the device. They will adequately protect your eyes and prevent any visual discomforts," Emma Williams assures us.

Summing up. With red light therapy, it's easy to do it right and hard to do it wrong, and either fail to get good results, or be unsafe. You can look forward to effective, non-invasive, safe results. "But there are simple and subtle mistakes that you can make that can reduce how effective your treatment is." What's most important is recognising these mistakes or missteps and avoiding, or correcting them, as soon as possible.

- It is also important that you pay close attention to how your body is being affected. Adapt and adjust your phototherapy regimens until you determine what works most effectively and comfortably for you.

- Red light and near-infrared therapy can become effective tools in helping you achieve your personal health and appearance goals, while you maintain complete control of your body and your sense of well-being.

Even more. We've covered quite a bit of ground so far, but there are a few things left to cover, notably bringing you up to speed on some other colours that may be used for certain types of phototherapies.

Chapter 7 - Even More Things You Need to Know

"The natural healing force within each one of us is the greatest force in getting well." — *Hippocrates*[8]

What Other Colours Are Used for Phototherapy?

This book is about everything you need to know regarding red light therapy, including its close neighbour on the spectrum—infrared light therapy. But what about the other visible colours of the spectrum; do any have beneficial qualities?

The specific effects and properties of visible light change within the range of wavelengths, which is one of the reasons why different colours of light are used for various light therapy applications.

We've touched on the two that are in use today for specialised applications; blue light and white light, and now we'll do a deeper dive into each, and follow with brief coverage of Violet, Indigo, Green, Yellow and Orange.

White Light Therapy

White light is a mixture of all the colours of the visible light spectrum. each of which corresponds to a specific wavelength range. It includes everything from violet, which has the shortest wavelength (around 400 nanometres), to red, which has the longest (around 700 nanometres). White light is an amalgamation

---

[8] Greek physician of the classical period

of red, orange, yellow, green, blue, indigo, and violet light. When all these colours combine, they appear white to the human eye. This phenomenon is most beautifully seen in a rainbow, where sunlight (white light) is refracted, or bent, and then dispersed or spread out by raindrops into the array of individual colours.

We've mentioned aspects of white light wavelengths in earlier chapters. Rounding out our review of various visible light colours—white light plays a unique role in healthcare. It's been found to be beneficial in combatting Seasonal Affective Disorder (SAD)—a type of depression that's associated with the shorter, darker days of autumn and winter. This therapeutic application of white light offers a ray of hope to those affected by this seasonal shift in mood.

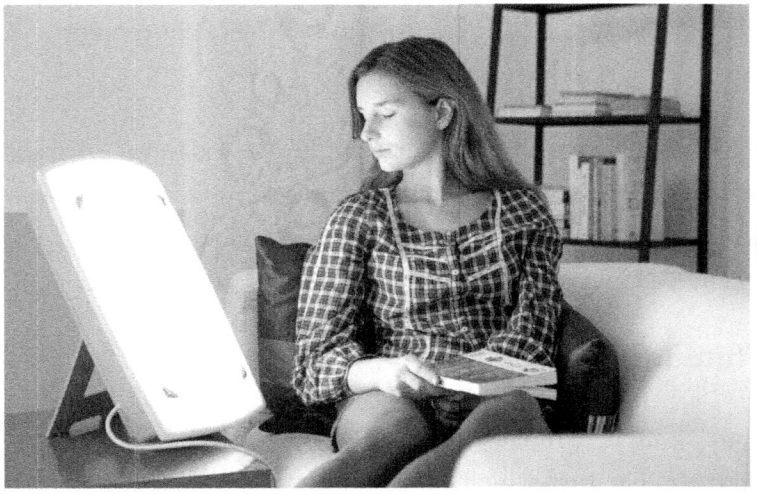

White light therapy is generally administered by a flat tabletop screen, often referred to as a white light therapy box. According to the Mayo Clinic (2022), the purpose of a white light therapy box is to mimic abundant outdoor light. "It's thought that this type of light may cause a chemical change in the brain that lifts your mood and eases other symptoms of SAD, such as being tired most of the time and sleeping too much."

Typically, a white light box should deliver an exposure of 10,000 lux of light while emitting minimal UV light—for obvious safety reasons. Check the packaging, which should indicate the light output and safety features.

Here is how and when to use the white light therapy box for best effects in avoiding and reducing SAD:

- The first hour after waking in the morning is ideal.

- Exposure should be about 20 to 30 minutes each day.

- Keep the light from 16 to 24 inches (41 to 61 centimetres) from your face, unless the instructions with the device recommend a different distance.

- You can keep your eyes open, but don't look directly at the light source.

White light boxes are widely available and are not expensive:

- Light boxes are not supervised or approved by the FDA for SAD treatment, so be sure to buy a reputable brand. There are many online sources, with a wide range of devices available in the $30 to $100 range. Amazon has many listings, as do other vendors.

- A light box can be purchased without a prescription, although your healthcare provider might suggest a particular model.

In summary, white light therapy should be a viable option for Seasonal Affective Order preventative and curative therapy, but is not otherwise applicable to other types of symptoms normally treated with light therapy.

Violet (Purple) Light

Purple light has the shortest wavelength of all visible light at around 380-450 nm. Some of these frequencies fall within the ultraviolet (UVA) range (315-400 nm). As we have discussed, UV can be harmful to skin and eyes with prolonged or intense exposure.

UV light has been used in certain medical applications, such as phototherapy for psoriasis and vitiligo, and in germicidal applications for its ability to kill bacteria and viruses. UV light is also used in fluorescent lamps where it is converted into visible light. These lamps are used in various applications, including phototherapy for Seasonal Affective Disorder, although the UV light itself is usually filtered out in much the same way as it is for light therapy products that use purple light. When used as a light therapy, purple light often combines the benefits of red and blue LED light, offering a unique blend of effects for various conditions—combatting acne while promoting skin rejuvenation.

Indigo (Cyan) Light

Indigo light, also sometimes referred to as turquoise or cyan light is somewhat nebulous in terms of its precise wavelength. In fact, indigo light is often omitted from simplified representations of the visible spectrum. The reasons for this are because the spectral bandwidth of indigo is not as wide as that of other colours. In addition, colour perception in this range can vary quite a lot between different individuals. However, the commonly cited ranges for indigo are around 420-450 nm.

Although there is limited scientific research specifically addressing the therapeutic benefits of indigo light, some potential applications have been explored:

- **Circadian Rhythm Regulation:** Indigo light is reported to be particularly effective in influencing our body's internal clock, or circadian rhythm as it is correctly called. One study suggested that indigo light could suppress the production of melatonin (a hormone that regulates sleep) more powerfully than light of other wavelengths. This would imply its potential use in managing sleep disorders.
- **Mood Disorders:** Light therapy, including the use of indigo light, has been used to treat SAD.
- **Skin Treatment:** Some preliminary studies and anecdotal evidence suggest that indigo light may have calming effects on the skin, helping to reduce inflammation and irritation.

Blue Light Therapy

Blue light falls within the wavelength range of about 450 to 495 nanometres on the visible light spectrum. You may have heard negative things about this wavelength: "Blue light from electronic devices gets a bad rap for straining eyes and disrupting sleep. But this natural wavelength of light isn't all bad," the Cleveland Clinic (2021) advises, and adds that "Blue light therapy can help clear up acne and treat sun damage and non-melanoma skin cancers."

Really, blue light can do that? You may even wonder why red light and near-infrared light have gotten all the attention, and blue light has been sitting quietly offstage. That's a fair question, so let's look into the issue of what blue light is for, and what it's not.

But just before we get started, you need to know that blue light therapy is best left in the hands of professionals; it's not a treatment you should be trying at home, even if there may be some blue light devices you get hold of.

Acne Treatment

Blue light is medically recognised as an effective treatment for certain types of acne. Many cases of common acne can be traced to a bacterium called Propionibacterium acnes, or P. acnes, which actually resides in oil glands that are just below the surface of your skin. By a fortuitous coincidence, P. acnes happens to emit its own photosensitizer, which means its receptors have a sensitivity to the wavelengths of blue light.

So, if blue light is directed toward acne-prone skin, at the right wavelength and the ideal intensity, it can wipe out the P. acnes bacteria and clear up the zits and blemishes. But it's not a guaranteed cure every time, because blue light therapy doesn't work for everybody, and some cases of acne are not caused by P. acnes.

If you receive blue light therapy for acne, it may take multiple sessions to learn if your acne is sensitive to blue light. Even if there is a response, and the acne begins to diminish, you may still need to use topical acne treatments, like prescription creams, or OTC (over the counter) products like benzoyl peroxide in Clearasil and many other brands. But for some whose skin responds, the treatment may be the ideal way to have clearer skin.

Blue light and near-infrared light therapies can be combined for further benefits: After the blue light treatment, near-infrared light therapy may be applied to cause the oil glands where the acne had been, to shrink in size. This dual action helps discourage further acne breakouts as it heals acne-caused skin damage.

Cancer Treatment

"Blue light treatment is most often used as part of a treatment called photodynamic therapy" notes Cleveland Clinic dermatologist Paul X. Benedetto, M.D., who explains the process and the benefits of this form of blue light therapy:

- Photodynamic therapy has the potential to reduce and eliminate certain kinds of skin cancer and precancerous spots called actinic keratoses, which are scaly, reddish, patches caused by extreme or long-term sun damage. Over time, they can become squamous cell carcinoma, a common type of skin cancer.

"To treat cancerous or precancerous spots with blue light phototherapy, a dermatologist first applies a photosensitizing medication to the skin," Dr. Benedetto explains. "That makes the treated area sensitive to damage by the blue light."

In the first, preliminary step, a specialised drug is applied to the skin and allowed to soak in for a specified time. Then the dermatologist directs blue light onto the treated skin for 15 minutes. The light destroys the cells that had absorbed the sensitising medication during the pretreatment. Several days after the blue light has been applied, the damaged cells have dried and risen to the surface of the skin or scalp, where it flakes off, leaving healthier, cancer-free, younger-looking skin.

"For the best results," Dr. Benedetto says, "You'll probably need to repeat the treatment two or three times, about four to six weeks apart."

Psoriasis

"Psoriasis is an autoimmune disease that causes thick skin with silvery scales that not only is unsightly but can be very itchy, too," reports *Woman and Wellness* (2022), noting that psoriasis is "Tough to treat, especially if it's widespread across the body."

In searching for new and more effective treatments, researchers and physicians are finding that the blue light wavelength appears to help reduce the appearance of psoriasis by preventing white blood cells from attacking the skin in an autoimmune response.

In a study published in 2012, both red and blue light therapy treatments were used in a test to treat psoriasis. Both light waves were effective, but the blue light provided a greater improvement in relieving the symptoms of psoriasis:

- "The clinical improvement of psoriasis, with respect to erythema, in particular after blue light and to a lesser extent after red light indicates that visible light treatment could represent a treatment option for psoriasis" (NIH/*Journal of the European Academy of Dermatology and Venereology*, 2011).

- The FDA, which rarely approves devices, did approve a wearable blue light device for mild psoriasis because multiple studies performed with the device showed the blue light significantly reduced or eliminated red and scaly patches while causing no side effects.

Summing up our study of "quiet phototherapy" blue light, it's best not to count it out for future increased awareness and application. We have to be impressed with the effectiveness blue light phototherapy is showing for acne treatment, non-invasive elimination of skin cancer, and effective results in treating psoriasis.

The extent to which blue light expands in usage will probably be limited by its availability to the general public, to purchase affordable devices for use at home. And blue light is not for everyone: Blue light therapy can be a problem for those who are sensitive to migraines. Our photoreceptors are more sensitive to blue light, which is why scientists believe blue light exposure can worsen migraine pain.

Add to this the concerns over the blue light from all of our digital devices, and it may not make sense to overload the public with a concentrated blue light on top of all this.

Finally, given concerns that blue light may not be as safe as red light therapy; let's leave it for the professionals to administer.

Green Light

Green light resides within the visible light spectrum with a wavelength ranging approximately from 500 to 565 nm. Green light serves a crucial role in various applications, from the photosynthesis process in plants, to specific kinds of light therapy in humans.

Unlike blue and white light therapies, there is not as much to say about green light therapy. It is believed that green light does not activate retinal pathways as much as other light rays, so it is less likely to induce a headache or migraine; reportedly, during a migraine attack, an individual is less prone to light sensitivity when exposed to green light. But there is little if any valid research to verify if green light lamps live up to claims of relieving migraines, and have been reported to increase, rather than reduce migraine pain in some cases.

There are green light lamps available online, but it may be better to head outdoors and spend some time in a green, natural, floral environment. This alone does appear to have some therapeutic benefits, especially stress reduction:

- Studies credit walking in natural settings, among trees, bushes, and grass, as conducive to stress reduction; the effusive presence of the colour green in nature probably has subtle therapeutic, relaxing qualities, in addition to whatever sounds and scents of nature add to the calming effect. This certainly works for me!

- The popular meditative approach to "being in the moment" or "mindfulness" raises awareness of what you see, hear, smell, and feel, and when performed in nature, is probably a worthwhile way to achieve inner peace.

Yellow Light

Yellow light occupies the segment of the visible light spectrum with wavelengths ranging roughly between 570 nm to 620 nm. Yellow light has unique characteristics that make it valuable in certain types of light therapy.

Specific scientific studies on the benefits of yellow light therapy are relatively limited compared to research on other wavelengths like red and near-infrared light. However, some studies suggest that yellow light therapy can offer potential benefits. Here are some of the proposed benefits based on early studies and anecdotal evidence:

- **Skin Health:** Yellow light therapy is often used in skincare due to its potential to stimulate collagen production, reduce redness, and improve overall skin tone. It is considered a good option for sensitive skin types that may react negatively to more aggressive therapies.

- **Wound Healing:** Some studies suggest that yellow light can promote wound healing and help reduce inflammation.

- **Mood Enhancement:** There is some evidence to suggest that yellow light can have mood-enhancing effects, although more research is needed in this area.

Orange Light

Orange light, a key part of the visible spectrum, has a wavelength that ranges from around 590 to 625 nm.

Orange light therapy, just like red and infrared light therapy, is a part of the broader category of photobiomodulation or low-level light therapy. Orange light falls in the middle of the visible light spectrum, and its effects on the human body are being studied. Some preliminary research suggests that it may aid in mood enhancement and energy balance.

Red Light Therapy and Botox

Botox and filler injections for skin care are defined as minimally invasive; they have become popular as a way to reduce wrinkles and expression lines as part of facial anti-ageing. "A report from the American Society of Plastic Surgeons from 2018 reported around 7.4 million injections of botulinum toxin (Botox) and 2.6 million dermal filler injections" were used that year, state Kaiyan Medical (2020).

Two questions arise relating to red light therapy and these treatments:

1. Those using Botox and fillers ask if red light therapy is safe to use after the injections, to relieve swelling and discomfort, and speed healing.

2. Those who are considering receiving Botox or filler injections ask if red light therapy is a viable alternative to help reduce fine lines and wrinkles.

There have been no extensive clinical trials to definitively answer these questions, but a consensus of dermatologists and skin care technicians suggests that red light therapy is safe and beneficial after the injections for most people, but each case needs medical oversight to ensure there are no side-effects or unexpected reactions.

As for choosing between the two options, there is no clear distinction; it's more a question of preference between the two approaches, with red light therapy being non-invasive but requiring a series of treatments, while Botox and fillers take effect more immediately, and the results last for months or longer after a single application.

Anyone considering Botox and fillers and/or red light therapy and has doubts and questions should meet and discuss these options with a medical practitioner.

Wrapping up. A brief conclusion is next, followed by a glossary of words and terms you may need to define, and finally, a list of all the links to articles and sources quoted in the book.

Julia E. Chatwin

Conclusion

"All that man needs for health and healing has been provided by God in nature, the Challenge of science is to find it."

— Paracelsus[9]

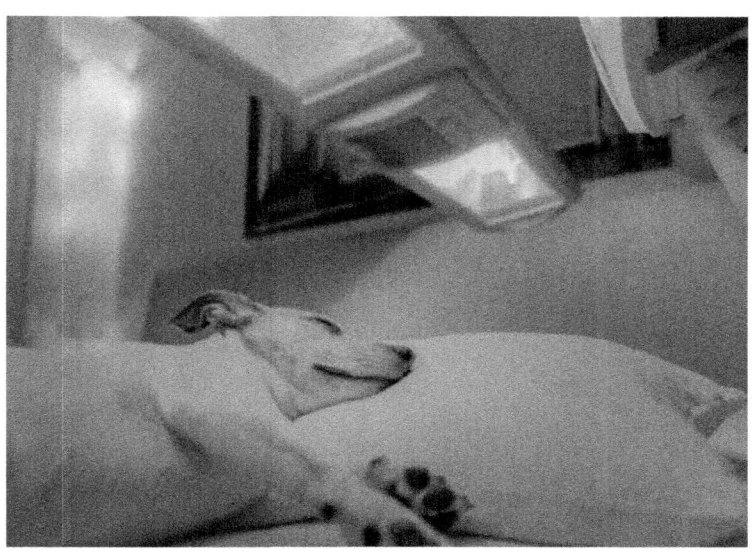

We've been on a journey of discovery together, learning about the science and personal applications of electromagnetic radiation—specifically the visible and near visible wavelengths of light. The light we see every day, sunlight, travels to us across 93 million miles of space. While red light, and near-infrared light, delivered by RLT devices reach us instantly from a distance measured in inches and centimetres. The effects of sunlight and light from an LED or laser light can have considerable differences:

---

[9] Swiss physician

- Sunlight is a composite of visible and non-visible wavelengths, some of which—red and near-infrared—are beneficial; some of which—UVA and UVB—can be dangerous.

- Red and near-infrared light emitted by LEDs, even in your home, is safe and beneficial, as long as the instructions for use are followed.

This is key: You don't have to risk sun damage to gain the positive benefits that sunlight provides. Red and near-infrared light can treat and condition your skin and body, safely, and relatively quickly.

We have seen that red light therapy is a promising therapeutic approach that has demonstrated numerous health benefits in various scientifically backed clinical studies. From reducing inflammation and pain, to promoting wound healing and enhancing skin health, its potential is huge. Moreover, its non-invasive nature and safety profile make it a suitable treatment option for a wide range of individuals with various health conditions.

While it is clear that further research is needed to fully understand the mechanisms behind the benefits of red light therapy, the existing evidence suggests that it is a powerful tool for improving health and well-being. As such, it is no surprise that this therapeutic approach is gaining popularity among health practitioners and individuals seeking non-invasive and effective treatments for various health conditions. This technology has the potential to transform healthcare in significant ways. Whether as a stand-alone therapy or in combination with other treatments, red light therapy is poised to become an essential tool for promoting health, healing, and vitality in individuals of all ages and backgrounds.

Finally, it is back to you. You have the choice of professionally administered red light and near-infrared therapy, or the more convenient and less costly home-based treatment with your own device. Just be sure to follow the guidelines in this book and buy the right device for you.

Remember the importance of medical care and counsel before you decide to begin. As Hippocrates reminds us, "First, do no harm."

Julia E. Chatwin

Glossary

Here, you will find a collection of key terms and definitions that will help you navigate the world of RLT. This glossary will serve as a valuable resource, clarifying the terminology that lies at the heart of this remarkable healing modality. The glossary also helps to reinforce knowledge and remind us of what has been covered.

Acne mask. Unlike screens of various sizes, certain red light therapy devices are designed for a specific treatment area. An acne mask fits over the face, allowing an internal array of LED lights to transmit the light directly to the skin where the acne and other facial blemishes are present. Unlike other devices, the LEDs, the source of the light therapy, are extremely close to the skin, necessitating very low power and intensity to avoid burn and overexposure. The light is not directed into the eyes, but goggles are strongly recommended for eye protection. Gloves are another type of highly localised application; LED lights inside the upper section treat age spots and other dark spots on the back of the hands.

Biostimulation: The process of using energy sources to stimulate biological activity.

Blue light. This wavelength has a distinctively mixed profile. We are exposed to blue light outdoors because it forms a large component of sunlight, and of course, it is the colour of the sky. Blue is also the colour of the light we stare at radiating from cell phones, computer and tablet screens, flat-screen LED televisions, LED indoor and outdoor lighting fixtures, and long-life fluorescent bulbs. Blue light is everywhere, and that can be a problem for those who are sensitive to migraines.

Cellular Metabolism: The set of chemical reactions that occur in living organisms in order to maintain life.

Circadian Rhythm: A natural, internal process that regulates the sleep-wake cycle and repeats roughly every 24 hours.

Collagen: The most abundant protein in the body, it provides structure to your skin, bones, tendons, and other body parts.

Dr. Endre Mester. A Hungarian physician and professor who in 1967 was the first to study how cancer cells react to electromagnetic radiation exposure, and to recognise that the newly invented laser had significant medical therapeutic value; that its intensity and precision could help to eradicate cancer cells. He later proved that low-level laser therapy could heal skin defects, burns, wounds, ulcers, and venous insufficiency. Venous insufficiency refers to a condition in which the veins, particularly in the legs, have difficulty returning blood back to the heart.

Dr. Niels Ryberg Finsen. A Faroe Islands/Icelandic physician is considered the father of modern light therapy, who began experimenting with light as a treatment for disease in the late 19th century. His theory of phototherapy stated that certain wavelengths of light have beneficial medical effects. Dr. Finsen was awarded the 1903 Nobel Prize in Medicine and Physiology.

Elastin: A protein in connective tissue that allows many tissues in the body to resume their shape after stretching or contracting.

Electromagnetic radiation (EMR) spectrum. The full range of wavelengths and frequencies, from the shortest wavelength to the longest. It is generally shown beginning on the left, with gamma rays and x-rays having the highest frequencies and shortest wavelengths; the spectrum then proceeds to the right with increasingly lower numbers of frequencies and longer wavelengths, culminating with microwaves and radio waves having the lowest frequencies and longest wavelengths:

Gamma Rays>X-Rays>UV Light>Visible Light>Infrared Light>Microwaves>Radio Waves

Green light. Green wavelength light possesses several therapeutic advantages compared to other visible light wavelengths. It has a lower likelihood of triggering headaches or migraines since it does not activate the retinal pathways as strongly.

Inflammation: A protective response involving immune cells, blood vessels, and molecular mediators to remove harmful stimuli.

Infrared (IR) Light: A type of radiant energy that's invisible to human eyes but can be felt as heat.

Joule (J): A unit of work or energy, equal to the work done by a force of one newton when its point of application moves one metre in the direction of action of the force.

Laser. The word is an acronym for Light Amplification by Stimulated Emission of Radiation. At low intensities, laser light waves can be therapeutic in phototherapy applications; at high intensities, it has many medical and industrial uses. The laser was invented in 1960 by American physicist Theodore H. Maiman.

LED. A light-emitting diode is a semiconductor device that releases visible light when an electric current passes through it. When electricity passes through an LED, the electrons recombine with holes (areas that are positively charged and created by the absence of electrons), and emit visible light, including the red and near-infrared light used in phototherapy, and at varying wavelengths for different levels of penetration. Chemicals are used to vary the colours of the light being emitted. Most red and near-infrared light devices used at home are based on LED lights; laser applications are primarily used in medical and other professional practices.

Light waves. Electromagnetic energy with two key characteristics: Frequency and Wavelength. Frequency is the number of oscillations of a wave per unit of time, measured in Hertz (Hz); wavelength is the distance between the two most near points in phase with each other. In other words, two adjacent peaks (or adjacent troughs) on a wave are separated by a distance of a single wavelength.

Mitochondria: The powerhouse of the cell, responsible for generating the energy that the cell (and body) needs to function.

Near-infrared light therapy (NIR): This is the next range of longer wavelengths on the spectrum, coming immediately after red, and is just beyond the range of visible colours. It is equally safe as red light, provides deeper subcutaneous penetration, and adds warmth energy, making it effective in treating sore and damaged muscles and joints. Certain devices allow NIR to be applied individually, or in combination with red light therapy.

Nitric oxide (NO): Also called nitrogen monoxide; it's a colourless gas formed by the oxidation of nitrogen, which performs important chemical signalling functions in humans and other animals. It is essential to the functioning of the mitochondria in our cells, functioning as both energy producers and metabolic regulators. Red and near-infrared light are absorbed by cytochrome c oxidase in the body, increasing the bioactivity of nitric oxide. This appears to return this enzyme's levels to normal, upregulating its activity while simultaneously enhancing energy production, cellular health, and general health.

Non-invasive: The term refers to a medical procedure that does not require entry into the body to achieve a result. It is therefore nonsurgical and does not involve the insertion of devices beneath the skin or into body openings. Light therapy, x-rays, CT (computerised tomography) and MRI (Magnetic Resonance Imaging) scans, ultrasound, and radiation therapy are examples of *non-invasive* treatments or tests. In addition to all forms of surgery, *invasive* procedures include endoscopy, angiogram, colonoscopy, cervical exam, and cystoscopy. All forms of phototherapy, including red and near-infrared, are non-invasive.

Oxidative Stress: An imbalance between free radicals and antioxidants in your body, which can lead to cell and tissue damage.

Photo bio-modulation: The beneficial impacts of red and near-infrared light therapy on muscles can be attributed to the stimulation of mitochondrial activity. This stimulation takes place when red or near-infrared photons, delivered to the tissue, are absorbed by cytochrome c oxidase. Muscles depend on adenosine triphosphate (ATP), the principal source of energy needed for muscle efforts. Thus, increased ATP levels are a recognised hypothesis to explain the beneficial effects that red light phototherapy has on muscle tissue. The slightly longer near-infrared light waves enable them to reach many of the muscle tissues and joints.

Photon: A particle representing a quantum of light or other electromagnetic radiation.

Photosensitivity: Although light therapy rarely causes side effects, some people may be photosensitive to light, due either to natural, or inherited causes, or possibly in reaction to medicines or supplements. If there is any possibility that a person has skin sensitivities to light (for example, hypersensitivity to sunlight), a skin sensitivity test is recommended before using a light therapy device. If a light therapy test, or starting regular use, finds that the skin is becoming excessively red, irritated or sensitive to touch, or itchy, it's best to stop the light therapy and give the skin a few days to return to normal. If the symptoms remain or return after resuming light therapy, it's time to stop exposing the skin to LED light and see your doctor.

Red light therapy (RLT): A type of phototherapy (treatment with a special type of light) that uses red low-level lasers or light-emitting diodes (LEDs) to treat various conditions, especially skin conditions. Red light is the longest wavelength and lowest frequency of the visible light colours of the spectrum.

Scientific Method: The standard way theories and hypotheses are tested for accuracy and validity.

Seasonal Affective Disorder (SAD): Changes in the seasons can cause changes in attitude and state of mind for some people. SAD is a type of depression, beginning in the fall and continuing as winter months grow colder and darker, draining energy and inducing a sense of moodiness. Phototherapy may provide relief, but not when treating skin disorders.

Side-effects: Most drugs, medicines, and treatments have been thoroughly tested and approved by medical authorities (like the FDA and CDC) before being administered by doctors or made available to the public at retail and online. But invariably some people will have unique reactions to otherwise safe treatments and may have symptoms such as rashes, dizziness, rapid heartbeat (tachycardia), diarrhoea, nausea, constipation, and gastritis, among others. To date, the consensus is that red and near-infrared light therapy do not cause side effects when used as directed. (See Photosensitivity.)

Spectrum. Isaac Newton's scientific experiments in 1667 with light and prisms led to a new understanding of the properties of light. By passing sunlight through prisms, which refracted (bent) the light, he was able to demonstrate that pure white sunlight was composed of seven visible colours: Red, orange, yellow, blue, green, indigo, and violet, which he called the light spectrum. We see the same effect in a rainbow.

UV Radiation. Ultraviolet is emitted from the sun in two forms: UVA and UVB, with varying positive and negative effects. Due to ultraviolet UVB light, prolonged exposure to sunlight can cause sunburn, skin dehydration (dryness), premature wrinkles, and most significantly, skin cancer. There are positive benefits from ultraviolet light in moderation, especially interacting with cholesterol in the skin to help form vitamin D3, which is essential for strong bones and to prevent osteoporosis.

Visible light. Your eye can see the light of wavelengths between 380 nm (shortest for violet) and 700 nm (longest for red). Although you can't see ultraviolet light, its UVA and UVB rays can burn or damage your skin; and while you can't see infrared light, you can feel its energy as warmth and heat. Infrared light extends from 700 nm (the wavelength where visible red ends) to 1,200 nm, the end of the therapeutic light window. (A nanometre or nm is one-billionth of a metre.)

Wavelength. See the light waves section above. Sunlight is composed of many different wavelengths, notably visible light, from red, orange, yellow, green, blue, indigo, to violet; it also contains infrared light, which is responsible for heat, and ultraviolet, which is composed of two types of rays, UVA and UVB, which helps form vitamin D, but is also responsible for sunburn, skin damage, and skin cancer (see UV Radiation, above).

Watt (W): The unit of power in the International System of Units (SI), equal to one joule per second.

Thank You

Thank you for choosing to spend your valuable time delving into the intricacies of red light therapy with me. I genuinely hope that the information and insights provided within these pages have enriched your understanding and will guide you in your journey towards improved health and wellbeing.

One small request, if I may: your opinions matter enormously, not just to me but also to potential future readers. If you found value in this book, would you be so kind as to share your thoughts in a quick review? Your insights and experiences can help others who are interested in exploring the world of red light therapy.

To write a few words about what you liked, what you learned, or how you plan to apply this knowledge, would be immensely appreciated.

Thank you once again for your time, your curiosity, and your desire to learn. It has been a privilege to accompany you on this journey.

To your health and well-being,

Julia E. Chatwin

About the Author

Julia Chatwin is an independent consultant and researcher. Her passion for a scientific approach to health and wellbeing is the driving force behind her literary contributions, manifesting in a desire to both deepen her own understanding, and enlighten others. An experienced author, Julia's prior success is exemplified by her bestselling book "DASH Diet for Beginners".

When not working or writing, Julia loves spending time with her family, cooking (especially baking), and walking her Jack Russell Terrier, called Tommy.

More Books by Julia E. Chatwin

If you enjoyed this guide book, you may also be interested in another book by the author:

DASH Diet for Beginners

Dietary Approaches to Stop Hypertension (DASH) is a heart-healthy eating plan designed to help lower blood pressure naturally. It is also a remarkable diet for weight loss and overall health. Available from Amazon.

Bibliography and References

The following sources and references have guided and supported the exploration of this fascinating subject and the creation of this book. Here, you will find academic research papers, scientific studies, reputable websites, and other relevant publications. I encourage you to explore these references further, delve deeper into specific topics, and gain a better perspective on the landscape of RLT beyond the confines of this book.

Alexander, H. (2019, June). *What's the difference between UVA and UVB rays?* M.D. Anderson Cancer Center. www.mdanderson.org/publications/focused-on-health/what-s-the-difference-between-uva-and-uvb-rays-.h15-1592991.html

Alzheimer's Society (UK). (2022). *Light therapy and dementia.* www.alzheimers.org.uk/about-dementia/treatments/alternative-therapies/light-therapy-and-dementia

Blundell, D. (2022, October 28). *Does red light therapy really work? Dermatologists explain the skin benefits. Women's Health.* www.womenshealthmag.com/beauty/a41409429/red-light-therapy/

Britannica. (2022). *Nitric oxide.* https://www.britannica.com/science/nitric-oxide

British Journal of Sports Medicine. (2006). *A randomized, placebo-controlled study of low light laser therapy.* https://www.ncbi.nlm.nih.gov/pmc/articles/PMC2491942/

Buyer's Guide. (2022, December, 2022). *Best red light therapy devices.* https://buyersguide.org/red-light-therapy-device/t/best?msclkid=ebb5c8a80af915ac7a81ab0366114dff&m=p&d=c&c=82807313796506&oid=kwd-82807905298480:loc-190&qs=different%20types%20of%20red%20light%20therapy&lp=93663&li=&nw=s&nts=1&tdid=10105779

Byju's. (2022). *Light emitting diodes (LED)*. https://byjus.com/physics/light-emitting-diode/

Byju's. (2022). *Relation between frequency and wavelength*. https://byjus.com/physics/frequency-and-wavelength/

Cleveland Clinic. (2022). *LED light therapy*. https://my.clevelandclinic.org/health/treatments/22146-led-light-therapy

Cleveland Clinic. (2022). *Red light therapy*. https://my.clevelandclinic.org/health/articles/22114-red-light-therapy

Cleveland Clinic. (2021, May 6). *Blue light therapy for the skin: What can it do?* https://health.clevelandclinic.org/blue-light-therapy-for-the-skin-what-can-it-do/

D'Abreu Chavez, M. E., et al. (2014, July-August). *Effects of low power light therapy on wound healing: LED x LASER*. ABD (NIH). https://www.ncbi.nlm.nih.gov/pmc/articles/PMC4148276/

DeAcetis, J. (2021, October 11). *The five best handheld LED light therapy devices for skincare*. Forbes. https://www.forbes.com/sites/josephdeacetis/2021/10/11/the-five-best-handheld-led-light-therapy-devices-for-skincare/?sh=396a6ace2c83

Dent, J. L. (2009). Professor Endre Mester: The father of photobiomodulation. *Laser Pain Therapy*. https://laserpaintherapy.com.au/wp-content/uploads/2017/10/Prof-Endre-Mester-Father-of-PBM.pdf

Dobrijevic, D. (2022, March 22). *The double-slit experiment: Is light a particle or a wave?* Space.com. https://www.space.com/double-slit-experiment-light-wave-or-particle

Doherty, C. (2021, May 19). Light: A therapy (and trigger) for migraines. Very Well Health.
https://www.verywellhealth.com/migraine-light-therapy-4114138

End All Disease. (2022). *History of red light therapy.* https://www.endalldisease.com/history-of-red-light-therapy/#The_Birth_of_the_LASER

Fadhel Al-Quisi, A., et al. (2019, May 6). *Efficacy of the LED Red Light Therapy in the treatment of temporomandibular disorders: Double blind randomized controlled trial.* National Institutes of Health (NIH). https://pubmed.ncbi.nlm.nih.gov/31205787/

Garibyan, L., et al. (2022 July 11). *Melasma: What are the best treatments?* Harvard Health Publishing. https://www.health.harvard.edu/blog/melasma-what-are-the-best-treatments-202207112776

Hamblin, M.R. (2019, September 6). *Photobiomodulation for the management of alopecia: mechanisms of action, patient selection and perspectives.* Dove Press. https://www.dovepress.com/photobiomodulation-for-the-management-of-alopecia-mechanisms-of-action-peer-reviewed-fulltext-article-CCID

Harvard Health Publishing (2019, October 1). *LED lights: Are they a cure for your skin woes?* https://www.health.harvard.edu/diseases-and-conditions/led-lights-are-they-a-cure-for-your-skin-woes

Hathaway, B. (2021, May 6). *How the skin's immune system cells coordinate defense against threats.* Yale News. https://news.yale.edu/2021/05/06/how-skins-immune-system-cells-coordinate-defense-against-threats

Higher Dose. (2022, July 15). *Red light therapy for thyroid: Everything you need to know.* https://higherdose.com/blogs/news/red-light-therapy-for-thyroid-everything-you-need-to-know

Johnson, J. (2019, July 29). *What to know about red light therapy.* Medical News Today.
https://www.medicalnewstoday.com/articles/325884#side-effects

Johnson, K. (2022, June 27). *Illumination the facts about red light therapy for sexual health*. Giddy. https://getmegiddy.com/red-light-therapy-sexual-health

Kaiyan Medical. (2020, December 19). *Light therapy: An alternative to Botox and fillers?* https://www.kaiyanmedical.com/post/light-therapy-an-alternative-to-botox-and-fillers

Kaiyan Medical. (2019, November 29). *Will red light therapy help melasma?* https://www.kaiyanmedical.com/post/will-red-light-therapy-help-melasma

Kleinpenning, M.M., et al. (2012, February 26). *Efficacy of blue light vs. red light in the treatment of psoriasis: a double-blind, randomized comparative study*. NIH National Library of Medicine. https://pubmed.ncbi.nlm.nih.gov/21435024/

Knight, J. (2022, November 13). *Does red light therapy cause side-effects?* Red Light Therapy Home. https://redlighttherapyhome.com/blogs/news/side-effects#What_Is_Red_Light_Therapy_Good_for_and_What_Are_Its_Side_Effects

Kubala, J. (2022, February 9). What is collagen and what is it good for? Healthline. https://www.healthline.com/nutrition/collagen

LED Aesthetics. (2022). *The benefits of yellow light therapy*. https://ledesthetics.com/blogs/science/benefits-of-yellow-light-therapy

Linde, A. (2022, December 1). *What are the benefits of red light therapy?* [Backed by science]. Therapeutic Beams. https://www.therapeuticbeams.com/red-light-therapy/benefits

Mayo Clinic. (2022). *Seasonal affective disorder (SAD)*. https://www.mayoclinic.org/diseases-conditions/seasonal-affective-disorder/diagnosis-treatment/drc-20364722

Mayo Clinic. (2022). *Seasonal Affective Disorder treatment: Choosing a white box*. https://www.mayoclinic.org/diseases-conditions/seasonal-affective-disorder/in-depth/seasonal-affective-disorder-treatment/art-20048298

McSween, D. (2022, November 10). *How to use red light therapy at home*. WikiHow. https://www.wikihow.com/Use-Red-Light-Therapy-at-Home

Mild, K. H., Mattsso, M., Hardell, L., Bowman, J. D., & Kundi, M. (2005). Occupational Carcinogens: ELF MFs. *Environmental Health Perspectives, 113*(11). https://doi.org/10.1289/ehp.113-1310936

NASA. (2022). *Regions of the electromagnetic spectrum*. https://imagine.gsfc.nasa.gov/science/toolbox/spectrum_chart.html

National Center for Biotechnology Information. (2018, April 19). *How does the thyroid gland work?* https://www.ncbi.nlm.nih.gov/books/NBK279388/#:~:text=The%20thyroid%20gland%20is%20a,thyroid%20hormones%20into%20the%20bloodstream.

National Center for Biotechnology Information. (2014, August 8). *Low level (light) therapy (LLLT) in skin: Stimulating, healing, restoring*. https://www.ncbi.nlm.nih.gov/pmc/articles/PMC4126803/

National Center for Biotechnology Information. (2016, December 9). *Photobiomodulation in human muscle tissue: An advantage in sports performance?* https://www.ncbi.nlm.nih.gov/pmc/articles/PMC5167494/

Nguyen, T. (2019, August 6). *Neutrogena recalls acne masks over concerns about blue light*. Chemical & Engineering News. https://cen.acs.org/safety/lab-safety/Neutrogena-recalls-acne-mask-over-concerns-about-blue-light/97/web/2019/08

NIH (National Institutes of Health (2016, April). *Killing cancer cells with the help of infrared light—Photoimmunotherapy*. https://www.cancer.gov/about-cancer/treatment/types/photoimmunotherapy-video

NIH (National Institutes of Health (2010, December 5). *Targeted light therapy destroys cancer cells*. https://www.nih.gov/news-events/nih-research-matters/targeted-light-therapy-destroys-cancer-cells

Pagán, C. (2021, November 29). *What is red light therapy?* WebMD. https://www.webmd.com/skin-problems-and-treatments/red-light-therapy

Omnilux LED. (2022). *Omnilux contour*. https://omniluxled.com/collections/all/products/omnilux-contour-glove

Platinum LED Therapy Lights. (2022, December). *The history of red light therapy*. https://platinumtherapylights.com/blogs/news/the-history-of-red-light-therapy

Platinum Therapy. (2021, July). *Ease your aches using red light therapy for pain*. https://platinumtherapylights.com/blogs/news/red-light-therapy-for-pain

Red Light Clinic. (2022). *Red light therapy research: Proven clinical studies*. https://redlightclinic.com/red-light-therapy-research-proven-clinical-studies/

Red Light Clinic. (2019, April 28. *Wavelength of red light*. https://redlightclinic.com/wavelength-of-red-light/

Red Light Man. (2022). *A history of light therapy*. https://redlightman.com/blog/history-light-therapy/

Red Light Therapy News. (2022). *All you need to know about red light therapy devices*. https://redlighttherapynews.com/devices/

Rouge Curve Commercial Red Light Therapy Unit. (n.d.). Rouge Care. Retrieved May 28, 2023, from https://rougecare.co.uk/products/rouge-curve-red-light-therapy-panel-on-motorized-stand

Smiley, J. (2022, March 17). *What is red light therapy?* Very Well Health. https://www.verywellhealth.com/red-light-therapy-5217767

Trivedi, M. K., et al. (2017, March). *A review of laser and LED therapy in melasma.* International Journal of Women's Dermatology. https://www.ncbi.nlm.nih.gov/pmc/articles/PMC5418955/

Trophy Skin. (2022). *Red light therapy and adverse side-effects.* https://trophyskin.com/pages/red-light-therapy-side-effects

Weiss, C. (2022, January 20). *Mayo Clinic Q & A: Light therapy for seasonal affective disorder.* Mayo Clinic. https://newsnetwork.mayoclinic.org/discussion/mayo-clinic-q-and-a-light-therapy-for-seasonal-affective-disorder/

WikiPedia. (2022). *Cytochrome_c_oxidase* https://en.wikipedia.org/wiki/Cytochrome_c_oxidase

WikiPedia. (2022). *Light therapy.* https://en.wikipedia.org/wiki/Light_therapy

WikiPedia. (2022). *Niels Ryberg Finsen.* https://en.wikipedia.org/wiki/Niels_Ryberg_Finsen

Williams, Emma. (2022, October 31). *13 Mistakes to avoid when using red light therapy at home.* Red Light Therapy News. https://redlighttherapynews.com/devices/tips-for-red-light-therapy-at-home/

Woman and Wellness. (2022), *Benefits of red and blue light therapy: Aging, acne and skin issues be gone!* https://womanandwellness.com/benefits-of-red-and-blue-light-therapy/

Wunsch, A., Matuschka, K. (2014, February 1). *A controlled trial to determine the efficacy of red and near-infrared light treatment in patient satisfaction, reduction of fine lines, wrinkles, skin roughness, and intradermal collagen density increase.*

Photomedicine and Laser Surgery (NIH). https://www.ncbi.nlm.nih.gov/pmc/articles/PMC3926176/

Yates, J. L. (2029, July 22). *Neutrogena recalls light therapy masks for risk of eye damage.* ABC 7 News. https://abc7news.com/neutrogena-light-therapy-mask-recall-recalled-for-risk-of-eye-damage/5410881/

Printed in Great Britain
by Amazon

26134627R00108